In Harmony with the Seasons

Herbs, Nutrition and Well-Being

Cathy McNease
The Herb Goddess of Ojai

MadeMark Publishing
New York City
www.mademarkpublishing.com

Cover Photograph by Bruce Ditchfield

ISBN: 069221514X
ISBN: 9780692215142

Other books co-authored by Cathy McNease

The Tao of Nutrition, 3rd Ed (with Maoshing Ni)

101 Vegetarian Delights (with Lily Chuang)

Table of Contents

Disclaimer   vii

Dedication   ix

Foreword   xi

Introduction   xiii

Harmonizing with the Seasons   xvii

I. — Spring   1

1. Allergies   3
2. A Rainbow of Foods   7
3. Eyes: A Window to Liver Health   10
4. Healing the Liver in Spring   14
5. Dampness, Phlegm and Fluids   16
6. Healing Our Troubled Hearts   18
7. Pain, Power and Peace   22
8. The Obesity Epidemic   24

II. — Summer   27

1. Spice Rack Medicinals   29
2. Treatment of Minor Injuries with Herbs and Foods   32
3. Medicinal Mushrooms: A True Super Food   35
4. Alcohol and Alcoholism   38

5. Sleep Troubles   40
6. Brain Health   44

III.— Fall   49

1. Gratitude Heals the Mind and Body   51
2. Breast Health   53
3. Indian Summer is Here   57
4. Lung Health in Autumn   59
5. Menopause and Other Middle Age Stresses   62
6. Sex and the Aging Woman   66

IV.— Winter   71

1. Dying at the New Year: Year of the Earth Rat   73
2. February: Heart Health Awareness Month   75
3. Inflammation: Causes and Cures   80
4. Kirin's Finger Is Saved!   83
5. Sugar: My Drug of Choice   85
6. Winter Solstice: Longer Days Are On the Way   89
7. Year of the Dragon: Chinese New Year   91
8. Pet Remedies   94
9. Tyler's 40 Day Vision Quest   98
10. Remembering My Parents   104

Appendix 1 Practitioners of Traditional Chinese Medicine   109
Appendix 2 Common Food Plant Families   139
Suggested Reading   145
About the Author   155

Disclaimer

THIS INFORMATION IS meant to inform, expand and provoke thought. If you are dealing with a serious health condition, seek proper medical attention. There are many qualified herbalists and Oriental Medicine practitioners across the country. The following sites may assist you in that quest for help:

http://www.americanherbalistsguild.com (Professional Herbalists)
http://www.nccaom.org (Practitioners of Acupuncture and Oriental Medicine)

Cathy McNease
Diplomate of Chinese Herbology (Dipl CH)
Registered Herbalist (RH), American Herbalist Guild

Dedication

My DEEP GRATITUDE goes to my brother, Mark, who has always been my best cheerleader and closest confidant. With his love, support, and technical skills, these articles are now available for everyone to read.

Foreword

I FIRST LEARNED about Cathy McNease through her association with Yo San University and the Ni family. I was hired to teach the Materia Medica classes that she had previously taught.

Her students introduced me to her skills in teaching herbal medicine with their stories. Cathy has a way of making the herbs come to life, including bringing in fresh samples of herbs from her garden. Her passion for Chinese medicine was infectious for these students, and she made the difficult task of learning many herb details a bit easier and a lot more fun.

Later, Cathy helped with the editing of my two herbal textbooks. Her attention to detail was very valuable. Additionally, *The Tao of Nutrition*, co-authored by Maoshing Ni and Cathy McNease, is a great source of information on dietary therapy. Cathy has the ability to simplify complex theories into practical information for both patients and students. She has been a great ambassador for the promotion of Traditional Chinese Medicine.

John K. Chen, Ph.D., Pharm.D., O.M.D., L.Ac.
Medical Consultant

Introduction

I HAVE BEEN fascinated by Nature and plants since I was a little girl in Indiana. Our family's downtown music business, that was also our home, was mostly surrounded by cement. It was the rich plant life along the borders and cracks of those parking lots that fascinated me. Outside my grandmother's piano teaching room was a sunny spot for Mullein to grow. Its soft leaves and tall stalks of butter yellow flowers seemed like perfect company for the day. Shepherd's Purse grew along the perimeter with peppery tasting seed pods, shaped like teeny little purses. The Dandelion flowers were my favorite. Mind you, I was only 6 or 7 and did not know that my playmates were actually medicinal plants. I discovered this much later when I transplanted my 24-year-old self to Southern California and bought Sky Heart Natural Foods. The logo was a winged heart, drawn from the Sufi symbol and the words of Kahil Gibran, *Awake at dawn with a winged heart and give thanks for another day of loving.*

With that, the course of my life as an herbalist had begun.

Sky Heart stocked around 100 herbs, along with all varieties of organic natural foods. This was 1975, so *organic foods* were not yet fashionable as today. Actually it was the accessibility of healthy foods in California that lured me from the natural foods wasteland in Indiana, where being a vegetarian was physically and emotionally very difficult. In California I began to learn from the old codgers who came into my store to buy herbs. I read every herb book I could find, old and new, and took many classes and seminars. Then, I got very sick and was unable to figure out how to help myself. Enter Traditional Chinese Medicine and the Taoist philosophy and world view.

My beloved partner at that time, Charlie, was a martial artist and lover of many Chinese traditions. He had begun going to acupuncture school in Santa Barbara and encouraged me to come meet his herb teacher. She was a medical doctor and herbalist from southern China. She and I immediately connected, and I went on to apprentice with her for 3 years. Now my feet were firmly placed on the path to becoming a skilled herbalist. Dr Jean Yu was a brilliant doctor and a very strict teacher, for which I thank my lucky stars. When she sold her clinic, the new doctor took me with the deal, so my next apprenticeship was with another brilliant herbalist from Beijing, Dr Henry Han. I interviewed all of his patients and explained the herbal formulas that he prescribed. This is the traditional way that ancient Chinese doctors passed on their craft, side by side with the student, in a clinical setting.

As Charlie and I were exploring Chinese herbs, we discovered the Ni family in Los Angeles. The father, Hua-Ching Ni, was in practice with his teenage sons, Maoshing and Daoshing, who were his apprentices. Meeting this family was another giant step along my path, physically, emotionally and professionally. My health was restored with a year of weekly acupuncture treatments in the Ni's clinic, daily bitter brews of Chinese herbs, and major dietary changes. This inspired me to learn more. The younger son, Maoshing Ni, offered a class in Chinese nutrition at their clinic. I was thrilled to learn about foods from a different angle. The extremism of the dietary dogmas, so prevalent in discussions at my store, made the common sense approach of Chinese nutrition refreshing. As it turns out, my notes taken at these classes were the beginning of the collaboration we created called *The Tao of Nutrition*.

Then, the matriarch of the family, Lily Chuang, asked me to assist her in teaching cooking classes and creating a cookbook, which we called *101 Vegetarian Delights*. Living and working around this incredible family of Taoist doctors changed me forever.

Teaching herbs and nutrition became my biggest love for the next 24 years. The Ni's school, Yo San University, and Santa Barbara College of Oriental Medicine, became my professional homes. Teaching, for me, was a lot like gardening. I planted the seeds in students' minds, then they cultivated the seeds (or not), and later would come back to show me their harvests. It gives me tremendous joy to realize how much healing has taken place in the offices of my former students over the decades. For that I am very proud.

One year at graduation, one of my Chinese students thanked me for preserving the medicine of his ancestors. That speaks to the reverence with which I practice and teach the body of medicine that has been passed on to me.

Now in my winter years, my focus has been on my patients, continually thrilled to witness the healing that herbs and lifestyle changes can create. I have the great good fortune to witness miracles on a regular basis. My goal is to provide a safe space for my patient to tell his or her story. Then, using the principles of diagnosis learned decades ago, I create an herbal formula and provide dietary guidance. Since I know that my patient will eat every day, the more I can influence their food choices, the deeper the healing will be. Hopefully, we will get to the root of the problem.

Growing plants, gathering seeds and watching Nature's cycles make my heart sing. Gardening and observing the life and death cycles of plants has given me much more patience, courage and peace as I watch the life cycles of my loved ones come to an end, as well as facing my own mortality. One of the first principles that I learned from my early Taoist teachers was that the cycles observed in the universe are a macrocosm of the same cycles observed in the human body. This was, after all, the way that the ancients first discovered the workings of Traditional Chinese Medicine...by watching the seasons change.

I heard a powerful lecture at the UCLA Medical School many years ago about Taoism by Dr Jeffrey Yuen, a very inspiring teacher. Taoists promote individual cultivation of one's spiritual life. Self improvement is taken very seriously. This puts all of the responsibility on the individual like that saying, *World peace begins with me.* Yuen's advice to the healer, is to live with wellness around you and people will be healed by your presence. Healing does not mean being disease-free. Healing means bringing the patient to the point that they want to make changes. This has been my life mission.

Nature heals. Thankfully, I discovered this fact in my youth and encourage everyone to breathe some fresh air, admire a tree, listen to the birds sing and smell the flowers. Nature is always there to embrace us as we gratefully bask in Her abundance.

Harmonizing with the Seasons

IMAGINE YOUR ENERGY is like that of a tree – if you observe the natural flow of the tree's energy through the seasons, you get an idea of being in harmony with Nature. In the winter the energy is deep in the trunk and roots, storing up for seasons to come. In spring the tree's energy moves upward and outward to the branches, forming buds. By summer the energy is at its peak of expression in the leaves, flowers and forming fruits. Late summer the fruits have formed and are becoming ripened, reflecting the tree's strongest concentration of life force. Contained in those fruits are the seeds for creating a whole new generation of trees. By autumn the tree's energy begins to recede into the large branches and trunk, causing the unsupported leaves to fall.

With Nature as our example of balance, we can adjust accordingly for better health and well-being, following the seasonal cycles. When our energy goes dramatically counter to this natural flow, we encounter health problems. For example, the excessive party behavior from November through January expends our energy, the opposite of storage - the net effect is high incidence of depression, anxiety and weakened immunity. A visit to the local farmers' market, not the supermarket, will get you in touch with the fruits and vegetables that are truly in season for your locale.

According the Traditional Chinese Medicine, the seasonal associations are as follows:

Spring – Liver/Gall Bladder (Wood Element)
Summer – Heart/Small Intestine (Fire Element)
Late Summer – Spleen/Pancreas/Stomach (Earth Element)
Autumn – Lungs/Large Intestine (Metal Element)
Winter – Kidneys/Bladder (Water Element)

Guidelines for Balance

Spring diet should nourish the Liver and help it to disperse stagnation, including plenty of dark leafy greens, sprouts, celery, lemon juice and green tea. Flax and sunflower seeds, mulberries and Gou Ji berries (Gou Qi Zi) will nourish the Liver. Light meats, legumes, whole grains and fruits round out the spring diet.

Movement is essential! Nothing will move your stagnation like exercise. Regulate sleep, with a goal of being asleep by 11:00 p.m. Late night eating or overeating interfere with restorative sleep and a healthy liver. Dandelion, milk thistle seed, turmeric, burdock and fennel all cleanse the Liver of toxicities.

Summer foods need to be light and easy to digest such as fruits, salads, grains and legumes, guarding against getting overheated AND overcooled. Both too much spicy food and too much cold raw food can lead to Summer time health problems. The goal is to stay cool and replenish fluids. Some bitter flavored greens can eliminate excess fluids and heat, often seen in swollen hands and feet in hot weather. Some spicy flavored herbs such as curry and peppers can open the pores, promote perspiration and cool the body, remembering that small amounts are balancing, while large amounts are harmful.

To prevent problems with summer heat and dehydration eat watermelon, cucumber, summer squash, tomato and lemon. Herbs to drink as cool, refreshing teas are peppermint, hibiscus, chrysanthemum and green tea.

Late summer is the transition season between the warmth of spring and summer and the coolness of fall and winter, and is associated with our digestive system. The diet must be easily digested – complex carbohydrates, whole grains, legumes, plenty of vegetables and some animal protein. Herbs to facilitate digestion are ginger, cardamom, fennel and anise seeds.

Autumn is the time that our energy is moving inward, the direction of the sour flavor. Foods like sourdough bread, yogurt, and sour fruits can help our energy to move inward. Begin to eat more warming foods and root vegetables. Seasonal fruits such as apples and pears can be prepared with warming spices like ginger and cinnamon. For those who tend towards dry cough or dry skin during this time may benefit from pears and pear juice. This is a time to let go of the past and work on forgiveness. Grief, contained in the Lungs, is often expressed now. Foods to strengthen the Lungs include fish, papaya, carrot, sweet potato, soymilk and almond. Herbs to strengthen the Lungs include astragalus (Huang Qi), codonopsis (Dang Shen), American ginseng (Xi Yang Shen) and lily bulb (Bai He), all available from an Oriental grocery. If phlegm tends to be your challenge, include garlic, ginger, cayenne, citrus peel, and all varieties of onions.

Winter is the time for storage, the time for conserving our energy and replenishing our reserves. Weak Kidney energy may present with a worsening of fears during this time of year. Exhaustion now is particularly harmful to the health, and may continue to be felt in the year to come. This is the time to be sure to get to bed early. Diet should focus on warming and strengthening the Kidneys, with a little more salty flavored food such as fish, seaweed, miso and tamari. Soups and stew are great for this season.

Warming and strengthening foods for winter include lamb, beef, chicken, turkey, salmon and trout, walnuts, chestnuts, garlic, black beans, oats, quinoa, cherries, dried fruits stewed with warming spices, and baked winter squash. Herbs for strengthening the Kidneys include Oriental ginseng (Ren Shen), cinnamon, dried ginger, cloves, and black sesame seeds.

So remember, our health, or lack thereof, probably began a season or two prior. Each meal is an opportunity for a healthier tomorrow! Begin today for a healthier year to come.

I.

Spring

Nature does not hurry, yet everything is accomplished. - Lao Tzu

CHAPTER 1

Allergies

HERE IN SOUTHERN California, many are plagued by allergies to pollens in the air. Extensive landscaping has turned a natural desert terrain into a lush, verdant landscape. As a result, we have an enormous variety of plant pollens to contend with. Typically, tree pollens cause spring time allergies, while herbs, grasses and flowers cause summer and fall allergies. Mold, mildew, dust, pet dander, feathers, cigarette smoke, and chemical pollutants, may all cause allergy symptoms year round, and can be difficult to diagnose. An allergic reaction is a disorder of the immune system that causes an over reaction to something in the environment. Anti-histamine drugs, like Benadryl or Claritin are used to reduce allergy symptoms.

Seasonal allergies to pollens can cause sneezing, runny nose, cough, asthma, itchy eyes, nose or ears; sore throat, hives, rashes and fatigue. Minimizing exposure to the offending pollens is advised, but that may be impossible to achieve. Allergic reactions can be mild or severe. If your parents suffered with hay fever (allergic rhinitis), eczema or allergic asthma, there is a good chance that you have inherited the "allergy-prone gene." From the point of view of Chinese Medicine, this shows an inherited weakness in the immune functions of both the Lungs and the Kidneys. Stress may be a trigger due to a the strong connection between the emotions and the immune system. Often the allergy-prone adult suffered allergies or eczema as a kid. Others may develop allergies later in life, even with no family history. Repeated exposure can be a trigger. Colds and allergies may have similar symptoms, but if those cold symptoms last more than a week, it may be due to allergies.

Several of my Santa Barbara patients have had to re-build portions of their homes after discovering extensive mold conditions. One of my patients reacted so strongly to the mold that it injured her intestines and she had to have a portion of her bowel removed. Another, after living next to the strawberry fields in Ventura for a couple of decades, developed a whole host of compromised immunity symptoms and neurological problems, as did both of her cats. The strawberry field workers wear hazmat suits when spreading fungicides and pesticides on the crops. I learned recently that part of the bee colony collapse is due to exposure to pesticides that have created a sort of "zombie bees" whose nervous systems have been so disrupted that they cannot fly home. All of us are exposed to chemical pollutants on a daily basis. For sensitive people, this may challenge the immune system to respond with a wide variety of symptoms. Respiratory and digestive complaints are common, as well as skin rashes. Sensitive patients may also be hyper sensitive to electromagnetic energies, cell phone towers, or chemical trails left by planes. Most of us are oblivious to these, but the sensitive person may suffer greatly.

For allergic children who have inherited this vulnerability in their immune systems, the following strategies may be of help to lessen their symptoms:

1. Identify allergens or triggers and keep them away from child (foods, chemicals, pets, pollens).
2. Hypo-allergenic lotions only; avoid lanolin and petroleum products. Stick with cotton clothing.
3. Breast feed babies. If a breast fed baby develops eczema, look at mom's diet for allergens.
4. Switch from cow's milk to goat's milk (or rice or almond milk for an older child).
5. Omega 3 Oils (from fish or flax) may help the skin and the immune system. Include beta-carotene rich foods, such as carrots, squash, pumpkin, greens and seaweeds. Mung bean and aduki bean soup may be helpful to clear dampness and heat (hot, moist rashes).

6. Watch for reactions to foods, especially: wheat, corn, eggs, shellfish, orange juice, bananas, peanuts, spicy foods, fermented foods, and pickled foods. Avoid fried foods, sweets, fruit juices and chocolate (this includes mom's diet if she is breastfeeding). Limit artificial flavors, colors, preservatives, and GMO (genetically modified) foods, as much as possible.

Food is another common cause of allergies, and these can be life threatening. I have a patient whose son was so severely allergic to peanuts that the smell of peanut butter from a classmate's sandwich was enough to send him into anaphylactic shock on two occasions. Allergy to gluten, the protein component in wheat, rye, barley, and their ancient cousins, spelt and kamut, causes a host of severe digestive complaints and can eventually injure the small intestines, leading to malnutrition. This allergy to gluten is called Celiac Disease. There is no cure but to avoid gluten containing foods. Nettle leaf tea and flax seed tea are suggested to restore the health of the small intestines in the Celiac patient.

A food allergy produces a whole body, immune response, visible in a blood panel. A food sensitivity causes a milder reaction to foods, without an immune response. Sensitivities can cause digestive complaints, bloating, joint pain and swelling. For example, someone who is allergic to milk gets cramps, pain and diarrhea when they consume it. Those who are just sensitive to dairy products may get mucus from them, but not severe symptoms. Some sensitivities may be due to the fact that the food is not appropriate for the body type. Milk is used to strengthen and moisten the body, but if you already tend to be strong and phlegmy, it is a poor choice. An experiment is easy to do, strictly avoiding the suspected food for 3 or 4 weeks, and observe how you feel. If the symptoms are mild, the problem food may be consumed occasionally. If severe, it ts best to avoid it all together.

When attempting to minimize allergic or sensitivity reactions to foods, it is suggested to rotate the offending food, no more frequently than every 5 days. Proteins are often the culprit in allergic reactions. Common ones are peanuts, tree nuts, shellfish, scale fish, dairy products, eggs, soybeans, and gluten (wheat protein). In the plant world, strawberries, tomatoes, mangoes, citrus, corn and mushrooms, are potential allergy triggers. With plant foods, it may be valuable to be aware of other foods in the same plant family. Sometimes the "cousins" can have similar chemistry and provoke reactions as well. Limiting the other members of the family may be suggested for those with severe food allergies. For more information, refer to "Appendix 2: Common Food Plant Families."

For dealing with the symptoms caused by airborne allergens, there are a number of helpful remedies. For both eye and nasal symptoms, I like to use *Pe Min Gan Wan*. It addresses the itchy, burning, watery eyes as well as the runny nose and sinus pressure. If it becomes a sinus infection with more pain and colored mucus, use *Bi Yan Pian*. If the allergies are either airborne or to foods, *Curing Pills* is a good remedy for acute digestive upset with nausea, vomiting or diarrhea. I also suggest *Curing Pills* for those who have sensitive digestion, easily upset by eating new foods, or stress. Another valuable Chinese remedy is *Yu Ping Feng San (Jade Wind Screen Powder)*. The primary herb, Astragalus (Huang Qi), strengthens the immunity of the respiratory system, building a "jade screen" to protect you from pathogens in the air. All of these are widely available in stores and online.

Quercetin, Bioflavinoids, Pantothenic Acid (a B vitamin), and vitamin C, are some of the supplements used to reduce allergic reactions, and control the histamine response. Another is Nettle leaf, which is made into tea or taken in capsules to reduce allergy symptoms. Ling Zhi (Ganoderma/Reishi mushroom) is one of my favorite remedies to regulate the immune system. It can be used both for a hyper-stimulated immune response as well as for a weakened immune system, and it is widely available in tinctures and tablets. There as a triplet of herbs: Ling Zhi (Ganoderma), Ku Shen (Sophora) and Gan Cao (Licorice), that has been extensively researched in China for the treatment of allergic asthma. They found that after 3 or 4 weeks of use, it reduced allergic asthma as well as the steroid treatments, but without the side effects. I use this formula for other immunity disorders, as well.

If you are suffering with allergies, find an herbalist to guide you. There is help.

CHAPTER 2

A Rainbow of Foods

I KNOW OF no better food advice for a long healthy life than to strive towards eating a rainbow of fruits and vegetables every day. Each color provides a power pack of nutrients to stave off chronic diseases and promote vitality. The USDA recently provided a new icon to represent a healthy diet, thanks to the work of Michelle Obama in attempting to raise food consciousness and tackle the childhood obesity epidemic. The image is a plate with ½ being devoted to fruits and vegetables, ¼ for proteins (lean meats, beans, eggs) and ¼ for grains (with the suggestion that at least ½ of the grains are whole grains). Off to the side is a small circle representing reduced fat dairy products (a glass of low fat milk or a container of yogurt). The brilliance is in its simplicity. Whether you are a child or a senior, you can understand the guidance. (Go to www.choosemyplate.gov for more dietary guidelines.) Most of us, even the healthiest of eaters, need to eat more fruits and vegetables. Reminding yourself of the rainbow helps move you towards that goal.

Red fruits and vegetables are colored by plant pigments called lycopene (in tomatoes, watermelon, pink grapefruit) or anthocyanins (in strawberries, cherries, raspberries, red grapes). Red foods protect our hearts, improve brain function, reduce the risk of osteoporosis and diabetes, and lower the risk of several cancers, most notably prostate cancer. In a study of men age 40 and older, those who consumed more than 10 servings of tomato products per week had two-thirds the risk of developing prostate cancer compared to those who ate less than 1.5 servings weekly. Lycopene in tomato paste is four times more bioavailable than that in fresh tomatoes, so ketchup counts.

Orange and yellow fruits and vegetables are colored by plant pigments called carotenoids. Studies show that these can help reduce the risk of cancer, heart disease and can improve immune system function. One study found that people who ate a diet rich in carotenoids were 43% less likely to develop age-related macular degeneration, an eye disorder common in the elderly, which can lead to blindness. Beta-carotene in sweet potatoes, pumpkins, winter squash, persimmons, papaya, peaches, and carrots, is converted to vitamin A which promotes healthy mucus membranes, protects the skin from UV radiation, helps prevent cataracts and exhibits anti-aging effects. Orange and yellow foods are also rich in vitamin C.

Yellow and green fruits and vegetables contain another group of carotenoids: lutein, zeaxanthin and xanthophylls. These are also important in preventing macular degeneration. You may choose spinach, broccoli, green beans, cabbage and corn for these nutrients.

Green fruits and vegetables are rich in folic acid and chlorophyll. Folic acid protects us from cancer, high levels of LDL (the bad cholesterol), regulates digestion and improves immune system function. All green foods also contain chlorophyll, nature's blood builder and detoxifier. The chlorophyll molecule and hemoglobin molecule (part of our blood) are almost identical in structure, except that magnesium is in the center of the chlorophyll while iron centers the hemoglobin. Thus, eating green foods is a very easy conversion for our bodies to make blood. In addition to all the leafy green vegetables, zucchini, peas and seaweeds, there are also a few green fruits: avocados, grapes, kiwis, limes and green apples.

Blue and purple foods contain a pigment called anthocyanins, the same pigment in some red foods. Grapes, eggplant, plums, blueberries, red cabbage, and beets are examples. This nutrient benefits the cardiovascular system, lowering cholesterol, helping maintain flexibility of blood vessels and supporting blood flow to the eyes and the nervous system. This may contribute to better visual acuity and reduction of glaucoma, as well as a reduced risk of cancer, stroke and heart disease. Reservatrol is another nutrient found primarily in the skin of grapes that may thwart a host of age related disorders including Alzheimer's disease. It has been shown to break down the plaque deposits that are so damaging to the brain. There are many studies showing a strong link between eating blueberries and improved memory and healthy aging.

White fruits and vegetables contain allicin, known to lower LDL (bad cholesterol) as well as blood pressure, and boost the immune system by stimulating natural killer B and T cells, the major regulators of the immune system defense. Examples are potatoes, onions, mushrooms, turnips, cauliflower, bananas, white peaches, and pears. These white foods also help reduce the risk of stomach cancer and heart disease. Bananas and potatoes are good sources of the mineral potassium.

We should all be eating at least 5 fist size portions of multi-colored fruits and vegetables every day. People who eat generous amounts of fruits and vegetables as part of a healthy diet are likely to reduce their risk of many chronic diseases. Did you eat your rainbow today?

For more information and research:
www.fruitsandveggiesmatter.gov
ewg@ewg.org (list of dirty dozen and clean 15 shopper's guide to pesticides in produce)
www.fruitsandveggiesmorematters.org

CHAPTER 3

Eyes: A Window to Liver Health

TRADITIONAL CHINESE MEDICINE has given us a way to physically view how healthy or unhealthy is our liver via the eyes. So much information is provided to me as a practitioner by simply observing my patient's eyes. The tongue is used in Chinese Medicine for diagnosis. The sides of the tongue tell you about liver health...pale = blood deficiency; red = heat; purple = stagnation. If your eyes are still in good condition, but you observe one of these colors on your tongue, start now to remedy the imbalance in your liver and protect your precious sense of vision. One of the beauties of tongue reading is that it empowers us to prevent diseases before they strike.

Here are some of the most important messages seen in the eyes, followed by some simple remedies:

Red eyes show heat, inflammation, or irritation.

Dry eyes show lack of body fluids, deficiency of blood or too much heat.

Itchy eyes show allergies, and the body's difficulty in clearing allergens. Nettle leaf, Milk thistle seed and Burdock root, all available in capsules, may be of help.

Watery eyes show inflammation. The extra tears are made in an attempt to soothe the irritation.

Sticky yellow discharge shows infection. A well strained tea made from Golden Seal, Coptis or Chamomile may provide relief as an eye wash.

Blurry vision may be a serious eye disease, so don't ignore this. It may also tell you that your liver is not getting the proper nourishment of colorful fruits and vegetables that it needs, leading to blood deficiency.

Pain in or around eyes may also be a serious disease, so don't delay in seeing a doctor if it persists. It may also signal stagnant energy or blood.

Floaters (floating flecks/squiggles in your vision) are usually due to a deficiency of blood, unless they appear all of a sudden; that could be a serious sign that needs medical attention immediately.

Dull, lifeless eyes show a serious mental-emotional disorder or severe stress. Guide this person to a professional for help.

REMEDIES:

For red, dry, inflamed, irritated eyes: reduce the amount of spicy foods consumed, especially raw garlic, coffee, alcohol and refined foods. These all heat up the liver and irritate the eyes. Peppermint, Chrysanthemum and Mulberry leaf tea would all be helpful internally. Apply a Peppermint tea bag to closed eyes for immediate relief. Another fabulous topical is to apply slices of cool cucumber for 10-15 minutes on closed eyelids. This has been a lifesaver for me in relieving eye pain from a cornea injury I sustained decades ago from my dog's paw. The cucumber remedy is also great after too much time staring at a computer screen.

For deficiency disorders (dryness, floaters, and blurry vision) some of the best foods will be green, orange and red fruits and vegetables. Spinach and collard greens are particularly high in the nutrients lutein and zeaxanthin which promote eye health. Carrots and sweet potatoes are rich in beta-carotene, another anti-oxidant that is important for eye health. Berries, cherries, and purple grapes are also loaded with eye nutrients. The popular Chinese food herb, Lycii berries (Gou Ji berries) are a delicious liver/blood/eye tonic. You can add them to oatmeal, trail mix or simple eat a small handful daily.

For pain and other stagnation eye problems: one of the very best foods is Bilberry. It is related to blueberry, which is a good second choice. Bilberry is available as a jam or a juice and is used to promote blood and oxygen flow into the eyes, as well as nourish and strengthen the blood vessels. During World War II it was observed that the British pilots had phenomenal night vision and an inquiry began as to why…it was the Bilberry jam that they ate daily on their English muffins! Bilberry has been shown to reduce risks of developing glaucoma, cataracts and macular degeneration. Increase your high fiber foods (beans, whole grains, fruits and vegetables) whenever stagnant energy or blood is your challenge. And, remember, nothing will move the blood like MOVEMENT!

For diminished visual acuity: think about doing some eye exercises. In high school I was determined not to wear glasses to read the black board. So I began to use a Tibetan eye chart daily for this, which was basically an elaborate mandala. As I followed the edges of the design with my eyes, it exercised them in all directions: up/ down, left/right, and multiple diagonals. It repaired my vision significantly and I did not require glasses again until I was in my late 40's. If your vision diminishes, consider a more nutrient dense diet to support the eyes, blood and liver.

Three of the most serious eye diseases affecting the aging population, all of which can eventually result in blindness, are glaucoma, macular degeneration and cataracts. Medical care is needed for all three; however, the progression of these diseases can be slowed down considerably with herbs and foods by nourishing the liver and improving circulation. You may also benefit from acupuncture treatments to further improve the blood flow into the eyes.

My guiding principles in suggesting diet changes for these patients would be as follows:

Glaucoma: reduce stagnation and include foods high in beta-carotene, Vitamins C and E, and sulfur: garlic, onions, beans, spinach, celery, turnips, yellow and orange veggies, green leafy veggies, seaweed, apples, oranges and tomatoes.

Macular degeneration: add to these bilberry, blueberry, kale and collards.

Cataract patients will also benefit from all of the above foods, but additionally, need to be very careful with toxins in the environment, smoking and sugar in the diet. Diabetics are at a much higher risk of developing cataracts.

Similason has a line of natural eye drops from Switzerland that I have found useful. They are available at drugstores and natural foods stores, with drops for various different eye problems. They are gentle but effective. For more food, herb and supplement suggestions for eye diseases refer to the following informative resources:

Natural Eye Care – An Encyclopedia: Complementary Treatments for Improving and Saving Your Eyes by Marc Grossman, OD, LAc. & Glen Swartwout, OD (ISBN 0-87983-704-7)

Healing Your Eyes with Chinese Medicine by Andy Rosenfarb, LAc. (ISBN-13:978-1-55643-662-8)

CHAPTER 4

Healing the Liver in Spring

SPRING HAS ARRIVED with its chirping baby birds, windy weather and multitudes of fragrant blossoms. The Spring is associated with the Wood Element (Liver and Gall Bladder). We will be the healthiest when we attempt to attune our energies to that of the natural seasons around us. Imagine your energy is like that of a tree - if you observe the natural flow of the tree's Qi (vital energy) through the seasons, you get an idea of being in harmony with Nature. In the winter the energy is deep in the trunk and roots, storing up for seasons to come. In spring the tree's Qi (vital energy) moves upward and outward to the branches, forming buds.

When our energy goes dramatically counter to this natural flow, we encounter health problems. In springtime if we are still indulging in the heavier winter storage fare, eating lots of meat, cheese and rich dishes, the end result is stagnant Liver Qi, allergies, headaches, skin conditions and lots of phlegm. A visit to the local farmers' market will get you in touch with the fruits and vegetables that are truly in season for your locale.

The following are guidelines for optimal health during this glorious spring season:

Our diet should nourish the Liver and help it to dispel and disperse stagnation and toxicity. This includes dark leafy greens, sprouts, celery, spinach, dandelion greens and green tea to cleanse the Liver and relieve stagnation. Lemon and lime juice clear Liver heat; flax, sunflower, pumpkin seeds and olive oil nourish the Liver, as well as poultry, legumes, whole grains, berries and fruits. This is a great time to be using Gou Qi Zi (Lycii berries) and Suan Zao Ren (Ziziphus seeds) to nourish the Liver blood. Green is the color associated with the Liver, so eating anything green, visualizing green and wearing green, will all benefit Liver health. And, avoiding artificial chemicals, preservatives, colorings, and trans fats, will reduce the burden placed on the functioning of the Liver. The Liver performs over 500 jobs daily for us...processing aspartame and red dye #2 should not have to be one of them.

The Liver needs movement!! Nothing will move your stagnation like exercise. Regulate sleep, with a goal of being asleep before the Wood (Liver-Gall Baldder) hours begin at 11 p.m., and no late night eating or overeating as this burdens the Liver's patent flow of Qi and contributes to stagnation of energy.

We know that the emotions associated with the Liver are anger, depression and frustration. On the positive side, this imbalance is resolved by practicing forgiveness. May we all seek to heal through the practice of forgiveness, especially now as we tune into spring.

CHAPTER 5

Dampness, Phlegm and Fluids

FLUID METABOLISM, ACCORDING to Traditional Chinese Medicine, is maintained primarily by three organ systems: Lung, Spleen and Kidney. Deep slow breathing will strengthen the Lungs. A gentle diet will benefit the Spleen and digestive system. Reducing stress and getting sufficient rest will maintain Kidney health.

Exercise is also an important factor in circulating the body fluids. When the normal body fluids do not properly circulate, they become turbid and accumulate to form pathological dampness or phlegm. That is the perfect environment for many pathogens to thrive such as yeast, fungi and bacteria.

Following are some foods that contribute to fluid increases or decreases.

Increased by:

– Refined flour products
– Refined sugar
– Sweets (even those made with natural sweeteners such as honey)
– Fried foods
– Dairy products
– Raw fruits and vegetables
– Too much salt

Decreased by:

– Whole, unrefined grains: especially basmati rice, barley, millet, rye, amaranth
– Bitter green vegetables such as bitter melon, endive, romaine, escarole, radicchio, arugula, mustard greens
– Celery, asparagus, bamboo shoots, pumpkin, turnips
– Beans: especially adzuki, mung, kidney
– All mushrooms
– Spices such as ginger, garlic, scallions, cumin, coriander, cardamom, fennel seeds
– Fiber foods such as oat bran, psyllium seed husks, apples
– Radishes
– Seaweeds, pears and almonds for respiratory phlegm
– Organic citrus peels made into tea (tangerine, orange, lemon, lime, grapefruit)
– Fish of all types
– Green tea and black tea

CHAPTER 6

Healing Our Troubled Hearts

STRESS KILLS. WE all know that to be a fact of life. But all of the emotions can injure us and cause sickness. According to Traditional Chinese Medicine (TCM), one of the major causes of physical disease are the emotions: anger, over-excitation, worry, sadness, grief, depression, fear and anxiety. Modern doctors would add to that injurious list: shame, guilt and resentments. There is a strong connection between the emotions and the immune system, born out in extensive scientific research. The Chinese say that holding resentments is like drinking poison and waiting for your enemy to die...ultimately we hurt ourselves by holding on.

According to the Theory of Five Elements, there are 5 energies that are observable in the environment. They are both changing and consistent over time. Each element has associated emotions that will affect the connected organs. They follow an order of generation like the seasons of the year:

Wood: Liver/Gall Bladder/Eyes
Anger, depression, frustration

Fire: Heart/Small Intestines/Pericardium
Over-excitation, over stimulation, anxiety

Earth: Spleen/Stomach/Pancreas (the digestive system)
Worry, over-thinking

Metal: Lung/Large Intestines/Skin
Sadness, grief

Water: Kidney/Bladder/Adrenals (endocrine and reproductive systems)
Fear, anxiety
The emotions are intended to be helpers...if we couldn't feel fear, we wouldn't be able to stay out of harm's way. BUT, when the emotions are either too extreme for the situation or too long standing...that is when illnesses can be triggered. If an organ system is weak or stagnant, it can contribute to emotional imbalances.

Similarly, the emotions over time can injure the associated organs. Here is an example of that. When sadness and grief are not appropriately processed and dealt with, commonly, the patient can develop lung or large intestine problems. I saw this years ago with a patient whose mother's death and her subsequent "emotional shut down" led to ten years of ER visits with life threatening asthma. Eventually, she took six months off from work to grieve. When she returned, the lungs were healed...no more asthma.

How do we heal the emotions? First, admit their existence and observe how they contribute to your life. What function do your emotions serve? Are they helping you or hurting you? We each heal emotions in different ways and on our own time line. Talking. Crying. Writing. Drawing. Creating. Exercising. Singing. Chanting. Meditating. Breathing. Prayer. Visualizations. For me, nothing works as well as Gratitude. Start and/or end every day with a mental list of 3 things you give thanks for. Over time this shifts your perception of what is really important.

As far as foods to calm the nervous system, nutrient dense, mineral-rich foods will be your best choice. Whole grains like brown rice, oats and quinoa are rich in the B vitamins and calcium; dark greens in any form, seaweeds, root vegetables – these are all mineral dense and high in magnesium. A calcium and/or magnesium supplement at night may help relax you into better sleep. Choose a digestible one. I have used the brand Rainbow Light for years. They have 3 Calcium-Magnesium food source supplements. Remember: calcium tightens the stool and magnesium loosens it, so a larger proportion of magnesium is stronger for relaxing muscle spasms, but can cause diarrhea. AND, avoid the inflaming foods: white flour and sugar, processed foods, trans-fats, animal fats, and fried foods. Physical inflammation can create emotional agitation.

There is a wonderful self-help book based on Chinese Medicine that I read years ago called, *Herbal Healing Secrets of the Orient*, written by an acupuncturist named Darlena L'Orange. In it she brilliantly laid out an expanded way to view the emotions which gives us direction in healing the unbalanced ones. On her chart called "5-Element Correspondences in TCM" she has the following included:

Wood:
Positive aspect: Enthusiasm
Task: Creativity
Resolve emotional imbalance: Forgiveness

Fire:
Positive aspect: Love
Task: Compassion
Resolve emotional imbalance: Surrender (ego)

Earth:
Positive aspect: Thoughtfulness
Task: Caring
Resolve emotional imbalance: Service

Metal:
Positive aspect: Spirituality
Task: Finding meaning
Resolve emotional imbalance: Companionship

Water:
Positive Aspect: Courage
Task: Finding inner strength
Resolve emotional imbalance: Faith

So for me, anger is usually my emotional issue. I tend to have imbalances with my Wood element, such as bitter taste, dry eyes, weak tendons/ligaments, and temporal headaches. *Forgiveness* is my path to resolve anger. If I can honor my *enthusiasm* and carry through with my task of expressing *creativity*, over time, my emotions will heal. World peace begins with me.

CHAPTER 7

Pain, Power and Peace

MY STORY WILL surely be a familiar one to anyone young at heart with an aging physical body. January in California is the time to prune the roses, cut back the dead of winter, and prepare the garden beds for the delights of spring plantings. For the past four decades, this is a time that has always garnered great inspiration for me with seed catalogs, gardening magazines and the hope of new life to come. This year was different...Early in the new year, after a weekend of what I thought was moderate yard work for my 61 year old frame, I injured my back and hip. The me of the past, post too much weed pulling, would take an Epsom salts bath, a cup of strong ginger tea (or some other analgesic herbs), take an aspirin or two and get a good night's sleep, and by morning I would be new again. This time, it didn't work. In fact, the pain progressed over three months until my nights were spent writhing on the floor with my legs up on a chair in the only position that provided any semblance of relief. Through this time I tried everything I knew: herbs, liniments, chiropractic, acupuncture, breathing exercises, heat/cold, restorative yoga, massage, processing emotions, calcium/magnesium, anti-inflammatory supplements such as turmeric and fish oil. Nothing changed. The pain was either going to break me or break me open, and mostly it seemed like the former was happening.

A couple of trips to my osteopath sent me in the direction of other medical specialists who provided Xrays, MRI, steroid injections into my back, pharmaceutics, narcotics, physical therapy sessions, and the pain persisted. What was I missing? I decided to try a different acupuncturist, a gentle and wise young Chinese man who I had trained in herbal medicine a decade prior, and my answer came. He made me feel safe and empowered so that healing could take place. On the first treatment, four needles were inserted along the side of my hip and leg. Tears poured, not from pain but from relief. When the treatment was done, I got off of his table pain free for the first time in three months! Since then, very mild pain has returned, but I am continuing with the healing treatments, including acupuncture, physical therapy, and herbs. I learned some new tools along the way that may be helpful to others with pain.

First, don't give up. Stay open to all possibilities, even from the strangest sources. The doctor who injected my spine only gave me a short break in the pain with the steroids, but provided a very necessary "mind shift" that will benefit me for the next decades of my life. He said that my weed pulling, hole digging days were over…"time to hire a young buck to do the heavy work, and save the fun and beautiful gardening for yourself." Instead of seeing my gardening days as over, they are just going to be modified for the new, older me. I don't have to give up my passion, just do it more wisely. He also suggested therapeutic pillows, including a body length pillow that goes between my legs at night to align my hip and spine and a cervical one that keeps my neck properly aligned. He suggested inverting myself with head below feet on a slant, and I have begun doing that daily on an inversion board, which gently stretches my compressed spine. The physical therapist has given me some simple exercises to stretch and build the tight muscles that are finally relaxing. Be open to the modifications necessary to stay healthy as you age. This may mean walking instead of running, fruit instead of cookies or rest instead of more coffee.

In the end, it looks like the pain broke me open to new possibilities and ways of enjoying my life in this 61 year old body, including having a handsome young buck now pulling my weeds, readying my garden for planting beautiful flowers. It's going to be a glorious Spring after all!

CHAPTER 8

The Obesity Epidemic

TODAY 2/3 OF adults and 1/3 of children are overweight or obese. Since the 1960's, the numbers have tripled! We are obsessed with dieting strategies, yet keep getting fatter and fatter. What's up with that? Obesity is quickly taking over the leading position that smoking has held for preventable deaths caused. Yet, we have such a hard time losing weight and keeping it off, even though it is killing us.

In the 1960's we began to hear about low fat foods for weight loss, but unfortunately this was not a good solution. The fats were substituted with refined carbohydrates. Then in the early 1970's high fructose corn syrup was created and became a cheap, sweet, food additive used in a huge proportion of prepared foods. This science project has a higher proportion of fructose than occurs in Nature, and our bodies end up converting it into fat. Unfortunately, our brain's pleasure areas are highly stimulated by these unhealthy foods, causing a true addiction to bad foods. Refined carbohydrates and unhealthy fats are highly addictive. The best carbohydrates are from vegetables, fruits, whole grains and beans. The healthy fats come from nuts, seeds, coconut, avocado, olive oil and fish. The worst fats are the hydrogenated oils or trans fats (another dangerous science project), which contribute to many diseases including heart disease and cancer.

Portion size is another big issue with weight loss/maintenance. If you realize that your stomach is about the size of your fist and can receive about the amount of food your open palms together could hold, that puts a huge meal into context. The best approach I have found is to emphasize non-starchy vegetables, fresh fruits and lean proteins; small amounts of whole grains, beans, seeds and nuts;

and stay away from the whites: flour, sugar and salt. Some people like to count fiber grams, aiming for 25-30 grams per day. That is a way to assure that you eat lots of vegies, fruits, whole grains and beans. The fiber helps to lower the blood sugar and maintain a full feeling. Beginning the meal with soup is another way to fill up on a low caloric dish before the more caloric main dish.

In recent decades with the technology boom, kids are no longer encouraged to go outside and play and instead are sitting and staring at a screen many hours of the day. It is essential to move more to lose weight. Getting into the habit of doing something active on a daily basis is one of the best strategies for health as well as weight loss. Walking, gardening, bicycling... find something fun to do, so you will do it regularly.

Waist size can be a useful measure of how bad our weight problem is: for a man, over 40" and for a woman, over 35", both signal a potential pre-diabetic imbalance. That "belly fat" is a killer, literally. It makes unhealthy hormones and contributes to heart disease, diabetes, and insatiable hunger. That is the reason that we pear shaped gals have a health advantage to the apple shaped bodies. Ultimately our goal is to reduce the belly fat, normalize hormones and regulate the blood sugar. This will all contribute to encouraging and maintaining weight loss.

Then, there is the whole "food as love/food as hate" issue when it comes to weight loss. I am from a family of multiple eating disorders. One of us nearly died many times due to anorexia nervosa. All of us have struggled with body image no matter what we weighed. Spotting the addictive trigger foods and strictly avoiding them is necessary for recovery. It may be foods that you are allergic to that you crave. Wheat, corn, dairy products and sugar are potential allergy causing foods to evaluate. Then, when you slip and eat that cake, learn to get back on your healthy path right away. Don't wait until Monday to resume your healthy habits. For getting in touch with the emotional reasons for overeating, and healing your relationship with food, I suggest the works of Geneen Roth, especially *Women, Food and God*. Clearly men suffer with eating disorders as well, but females still greatly out number the males in our culture of glamorizing thinness.

Ear acupuncture may help curb cravings in the beginning. Julia Ross' book, *The Diet Cure*, provides some supplements and amino acids that may help your journey as well. The Chinese would encourage you to use herbs to strengthen the digestive system to make it function more efficiently, thus normalizing appetite and weight. Fennel seed or anise seed tea is useful as a regular beverage to reduce the appetite and promote digestion. A probiotic supplement first thing in the morning may be another beneficial tool to improve digestion. Have you tried the delicious, low calorie, probiotic beverages from the Ventura, California, based company, KeVita, recently named as one of the 25 most innovative consumer products by Forbes.com. Look for them wherever they sell fresh juices.

Michael Pollan's sage advice from *In Defense of Food* is poignantly simple: "Eat food. Not too much. Mostly plants."

REFERENCES:

Ultra-Metabolism by Mark Hyman, MD. This provides a simple, whole foods approach to weight loss, utilizing foods to regulate the blood sugar and promote health.

The Diet Cure by Julia Ross, MA. This looks at brain chemistry contributions to food cravings, weight problems and mood swings.

Releasing Fat by Ray D Strand, MD. Explores living a healthier lifestyle for permanent weight loss by managing blood sugar and making wise food choices.

Food Rules by Michael Pollan. Simple ways to think about foods and eating responsibly for your health and the health of the planet.

Women, Food and God by Geneen Roth. She has pioneered ways to develop a healthy relationship with food.

II.

Summer

Eat food. Mostly plants. Not too much. - Michael Pollan

CHAPTER 1

Spice Rack Medicinals

MANY POWERFUL MEDICINES from around the world are currently in your kitchen pantry. I am talking about those flavor-enhancing herbs and spices. They are potent for many acute and chronic health complaints. For chronic conditions, consider using them regularly in your food; for acute conditions you can make a cup of tea by steeping ½ - 1 teaspoon of the crushed herb or spice with a pint of boiling water. Let it soak about 10-15 minutes, then strain and drink in 2 or 3 portions throughout the day.

Digestive and Urinary Aids

Seeds of Anise, Fennel, Cardomom, Caraway, Dill, Coriander (Cilantro seeds), Cumin – all improve digestion, relieving discomfort, indigestion, bloating and gas. The tea will be stronger if seeds are crushed in your mortar and pestle or coffee grinder before preparing. **Parsley** promotes digestion, especially if you overeat. Additionally, **Parsley** promotes urination to reduce edema and strengthens the kidneys and adrenals. **Celery seeds** will relieve water swelling and the pain of gout. **Sesame, Hemp and Flax seeds** ease constipation. **Ginger** and **Cinnamon** aid chronic diarrhea, especially when cooked into a white rice porridge (lots of water, not much rice, cooked for 1 hour).

Pain Relief

Ginger, Cinnamon, Cloves, Allspice all help warm the circulation. Think about the mulling spice mixes that we use with apple cider in autumn...this group are great for pain. A painful tooth can be numbed by holding a whole **Clove** in your mouth near the problem tooth.

Cayenne pepper – its heat can improve blood flow to painful areas with just a pinch. Apply to cuts to stop bleeding quickly. Put in socks to keep feet warm. Capsaisin pain ointments are derived from this spice and used for shingles topically.

Turmeric is a powerful anti-inflammatory, used for liver, gall bladder and stomach conditions, as well as joint pain. In India, this is eaten daily in curries and their incidence of dementia is very low as a result. Indians also apply it to cuts, rashes and sores. Curcumin, the active ingredient, is available in supplement form. (Not for those on blood thinning drugs.)

Saffron is a powerful blood moving herb...only a few threads at a time are needed. This helps pain anywhere in the body due to poor circulation. (Not for those on blood thinning drugs.)

Rosemary and **Peppermint** are both good teas for headaches and sinus pain. **Peppermint** is not for GERD patients because it relaxes the stomach sphincter, allowing for the upward acid movement that causes heartburn, chronic cough and chronic throat discomfort. (Although not a cooking herb, **Slippery Elm Bark** tea may help heal that inflamed stomach.)

Colds and Respiratory Problems

Basil, Cilantro (Coriander leaves), Scallions, Perilla, Ginger, Garlic, Sage, Thyme: these all have anti-viral, anti-bacterial properties to help hasten the healing of a respiratory infection.

Sage and **Thyme** will be particularly drying for cases with lots of phlegm discharge.

Systemic Infections

Garlic has a wide reputation as "poor man's penicillin", treating virus, bacteria, parasites, fungus and yeast; it improves heart health and circulation. (Not good for those with dry eyes or mouth sores.)

Oregano is equally powerful for fungal and bacterial infections. Sprinkle on food daily to prevent illness and assist the immune system. Cousin **Marjoram** is similar, but milder.

Fresh Ginger Root is especially effective with digestive "bugs" causing nausea, vomiting, diarrhea, indigestion, and for the treatment of food poisoning.

CHAPTER 2

Treatment of Minor Injuries with Herbs and Foods

SUMMER TIME FINDS us spending more time outside at play in the long days, and sometimes that leads to an injury. Many simple home remedies can alleviate suffering. What follows are some simple remedies to help with the booboos of summer. Once the very hot days arrive, watermelon, tomatoes, cucumbers, summer squash, lemon juice and mung beans, can all be used to prevent dehydration and overheating. A large natural food store or Oriental market will have all of the remedies mentioned.

Simple Herbal Home Remedies for Common Ailments

Abdominal pain: valerian; chamomile; fennel; ginger; cinnamon; peony + licorice

Anxiety: valerian; chamomile; poppy; passion flower vine; Cal-Mag;

Bee stings: clay; plantain; aloe; vinegar + baking soda

Bladder infection: uva ursi; marshmallow; dandelion; cranberry; coptis; D-Mannose

Bleeding: tienchi; comfrey root powder; cayenne; seaweed; yarrow; charcoal

Bruises: tienchi; turmeric; Zheng Gu Shui liniment; fresh ginger poultice; arnica ointment

Boils: clay; dandelion; honeysuckle; coptis; goldenseal; violet leaf

Burns: honey; aloe; calendula; lavender oil; Ching Wan Hung burn ointment

Colds: Fever more- mint, echinacea; lemon balm; feverfew; honeysuckle; Yin Qiao

Chills more- fresh ginger, garlic, cayenne;

Cold sores (herpes simplex): isatis leaf or root; lemon balm (melissa); tree tree oil

Colic: fennel; ginger; catnip; chamomile; mint

Constipation: honey; olive oil; aloe gel; Triphala; flax seeds; psyllium husks (+water)

Cough: eucalyptus oil (steam), ginger; garlic; licorice; mullein, marshmallow root; apricot seeds; honey (dry cough); pears; Planetary Old Indian Syrup

Cuts: tienchi; calendula; comfrey; dandelion; plantain; coptis; goldenseal

Diarrhea: white rice; pectin; probiotics; black tea; blackberry or raspberry leaf; Huang Lian Su Pian; kudzu; if watery and cold- Chinese yam, cinnamon; if hot and burning- slippery elm

Dysmenorrhea: valerian; turmeric; ginger; saffron; dang gui; peony; motherwort

Earache: mullein oil; garlic oil; echinacea; Bi Yan Pian

Fever: feverfew; mint; elder; honeysuckle; echinacea; lemon balm; Yin Qiao; Vit.C; if due to weakness-American Ginseng

Flu: see "colds": boneset; Arnica oil (for massage); Oscillococcinum; isatis

Food poisoning: honeysuckle; fresh ginger; perilla; garlic; charcoal; Huo Xiang Zheng Qi Wan (also for stomach flu); Huang Lian Su Pian

Fungal infection: pau d'arco; tea tree oil; Citricidal; vinegar; thyme

Hangover: mung bean; shen qu; umeboshi-kudzu broth; pears; B vitamins; water

Headache: Chuan Xiong Cha Tiao Wan; feverfew; White Flower Oil; peppermint

Heartburn: goldenseal; Huang Lian Su; cuttlefish bone; DGL licorice tablets; slippery elm

Indigestion: chamomile; mint; hawthorn; papaya; Curing Pills; umeboshi plum

Insomnia: chamomile; valerian; scullcap; Suan Zao Ren Tang; Cal-Mag; passion flower vine; hops; Planetary Herbal's Valerian Easy Sleep

Liver injury by Tylenol: prevent with burdock root; milk thistle seed

Nausea: fresh ginger; chamomile; mint; Huo Xiang Zheng Qi Wan/Shui

Nerve pain (tooth, smashed finger, stubbed toe): St. John's wort oil, tincture, or homeopathic (Contraindicated with many pharmaceuticals including birth control pills, anti-depressants, chemotherapy drugs and blood thinners)

Parasites: garlic; pumpkin seeds; walnut husks; wormwood; Citricidal

PMS: Xiao Yao Wan; chasteberry; peony; cyperus; Cal-Mag

Poison Oak: mugwort; clay; dandelion; calendula; Yin Qiao; vinegar; oatmeal baths; Xiao Feng San; plantain leaf; jewelweed

Shock: 911!; Rescue Remedy; if limbs are limp and cold- ginger, ginseng, cayenne

Sores: calendula; comfrey; plantain; tea tree oil; coptis; goldenseal; Manuka honey

Spider bites: charcoal paste; coptis; golden seal; plantain; vinegar + baking soda

Staph/Strep infections: tea tree oil; echinacea; garlic; lavender oil; coptis; Manuka honey; Citricidal

Throat pain: licorice; mint; burdock; salt water gargle; isatis root/leaf; Yin Qiao

Vaccination reactions: echinacea; Thuja (homeopathic)

Vaginal infections: tea tree oil; Citricidal; white vinegar (not cider); Yin Care

Viral infections: echinacea; ginger; honeysuckle; Citricidal; garlic; Yin Qiao; isatis root or leaf

Vomiting: fresh ginger; mint; chamomile; Huo Xiang Zheng Qi Wan

Wounds: calendula; comfrey; tienchi; dandelion

Yeast infections: tea tree oil; Citricidal; pau d'arco; garlic; probiotics

Please note that these remedies are provided as educational and anecdotal information and are not intended to replace care by a medical professional. If a simple ailment does not improve in a short amount of time, more specific diagnostics may be indicated.

CHAPTER 3

Medicinal Mushrooms: A True Super Food

I FIRST SAW medicinal mushrooms being used in a family of Taoist healers with whom I was apprenticing in the early 1980's. I had been asked to help the matriarch teach cooking classes, since she spoke very little English. Lily Chuang was a brilliant herbalist, but she preferred to prevent illnesses in her family rather than treat them. One of the tricks up her sleeve was regular use of **Shitake Mushrooms** (Lentinula edodes). She always had a jar of the dried mushrooms rehydrating in the refrigerator. Every meal included a small amount of these gems, cooked with eggs, in oatmeal, in soups and stir fries. She even made "burgers" out of the tough dry stems that she powdered in a coffee grinder and mixed with grated vegetables and eggs, and pan fried until brown. The soaking water from the rehydration process was used as a delicious addition to soups and grains.

Nowadays, **Shitakes** are widely available in many forms-dried, fresh in the produce section and incorporated into capsules and tablets of medicinal mushroom blends. Shitakes are one of the most flavorful mushrooms to use as food, while some of the others are too bitter or woody to use this way, and are better taken in capsule form. Shitake mushrooms are very rich in a large sugar molecule called a polysaccharide, which has been found to show strong anti-tumor, anti-viral and immune enhancing effects, such as increasing macrophage and killer T-cell activity. Shitakes have been shown to improve the health of chronic hepatitis, HIV and AIDS patients. Research also has shown their ability to lower both blood pressure and cholesterol. General dosage as food would be to eat 2-5 mushrooms daily, cooked in some form (or taken as directed in capsules). **Maitake** (Grifola frondosa), another delicious mushroom, but not as widely available, has been found to be even stronger in its action against cancer.

Two other woody textured medicinal mushrooms that are powerful healers are not eaten as foods, but taken in teas, tablets or capsules: **Chaga** (Inonotus obliquus)** and **Ganoderma Lucidum** (aka Reishi, Ling Zhi). Chaga has long been used in Russia and Eastern Europe for treatment of cancers, gastritis and stomach ulcers. It has an enormously high level of anti-oxidants for reducing inflammation, fighting infections and promoting good health. Chaga is available from Canadian suppliers in a powdered form which can be prepared as a pleasant tea (www.mitobi.com). With cancer on both sides of my family, this tea has become one of my staples.

Ganoderma Mushroom is used as an immune-modulator, which means that it normalizes both an overactive immune system (auto-immune conditions) and an underactive immune system (frequent or chronic infections). It is not generally used as a tea due to the bitter flavor, but is widely available in pills, capsules and tinctures (alcohol extracts). Ganoderma has been used in the Chinese pharmacopoeia for over 3,000 years. Its benefits include: anti-inflammatory, liver protective, anti-tumor, reducing altitude sickness (by improved oxygen utilization), anti-histamine, cholesterol lowering, and lowering of mental disease symptoms caused by environmental stress. With older patients, the research shows a marked benefit on the heart and lungs in conditions such as coronary artery disease, palpitations, dyspnea (difficulty breathing) and chronic bronchitis.

One of the most restorative mushrooms from the Chinese tradition is actually a combination of a fungus and a caterpillar: **Cordyceps** (Dong Chong Xia Cao=Winter Worm Summer Grass). This is a caterpillar that freezes just under the surface of the ground in winter, and in spring a fungus grows out from its body. These are very expensive and are now being cultivated minus the caterpillar. This is considered in Chinese medicine to be a very powerful, deeply strengthening immune tonic, used in serious problems such as bone marrow failure, HIV-AIDS, Chronic Fatigue Syndrome and generalized weakness. They were made famous recently when a group of very successful Chinese female athletes credited their Olympic success to **Cordyceps**. They are often included in the medicinal mushroom blends that are prepared into capsules and available at your local health food stores. In traditional Chinese culture, **Cordyceps** are prepared into meat and poultry soups with other herbs like ginseng. A word to the wise…if you do this, crush up the **Cordyceps** first; otherwise, when it re-hydrates into the soup, the caterpillar clearly become visible and may be staring back at you on your soup spoon.

For further information and research details, go to the following sites:

www.christopherhobbs.com
www.drweil.com
http://www.fungi.com

**Instructions for preparing Chaga tea:

Put 2 tablespoons of the powdered chaga mushrooms in a non-aluminum, non-Teflon pan with 3-4 cups of pure water. Cover and simmer for 20-30 minutes. Strain off the tea and do a second boiling with another 3-4 cups of pure water, again simmering for 20-30 minutes. Strain the tea and combine with the first boiling. Refrigerate and reheat before drinking. This will last a week in the refrigerator. Drink 1-3 cups of tea per day.

CHAPTER 4

Alcohol and Alcoholism

MOST FAMILIES HAVE alcoholics among us. We often see the genetic component manifest with heartbreaking stories. One of my patients who is 38, got sober 2 years ago because his father and 3 uncles all died in their late 30's from complications of alcoholism. For those with the genes that cannot handle alcohol, drinking is not a choice. Unfortunately we live in a culture that encourages drinking and is not very tolerate of we teetotalers.

From the point of view of Chinese medicine, all alcoholic drinks are very warming in nature. That is one of the big problems it creates in excess quantities...dehydration. The B vitamin complex is depleted, and internal heat and inflammation is created or worsened. I rarely drink alcohol, but if I do, the night always ends with a B vitamin complex, Milk Thistle capsules and a tall glass of water. This reduces the hangover discomfort the next day.

Long term alcoholism is associated with serious health consequences. Its toxic effect on the nervous system can lead to depression and other psychological problems. It increases risk of high blood pressure, erectile dysfunction, stroke, several types of cancers, and eventually, long term, there will be brain damage, liver damage and kidney disease. It's grim.

Recommendations:

Stop all alcohol.

Daily eat several servings of green, orange or yellow vegies, all high in vitamin A to reduce cravings and heal the liver.

Eat adequate protein to maintain weight and normal brain functioning. Fish, eggs, dairy foods are all great choices.

Kudzu root and flower for cravings

Fish oil caps, amino acids and 5HTP for depression

Milk thistle seed or the active ingredient, silymarin, in capsules for repairing the liver

Reishi or Ganoderma mushroom to prevent fatty liver and cirrhosis

Take a multiple vitamin and mineral tablet with a good dose of the B vitamins

Chapter 5

Sleep Troubles

INSOMNIA, HYPERTENSION AND restless mind can all come down to an imbalance in Yin and Yang. Yin is like water, cool and calming. Yang is like fire, hot and activating. When we have insufficient Yin to balance that excessive Yang, many uncomfortable and dangerous symptoms ensue. Stress agitates us and dries up our Yin. Bad diet inflames us and increases our Yang. Women become deficient in Yin very often thanks to our menstrual cycles. By the end of our busy days, we are really depleted of Yin, so bedtime rolls around and either the mind is so busy we can't even close our eyes, or we fall into sleep, only to awaken in a short time feeling restless. Be sure to stay hydrated all day, our first way of restoring Yin.

The goal then becomes preserving the Yin and controlling the Yang. I love to take a beach break in my mind with the following visualization. Imagine that your feet are at the edge of the ocean or standing in cool, moist grass. Inhale through the bottoms of the feet, bringing that cool Yin energy up to your belly. Then exhale down your legs through the bottoms of the feet, releasing all of the hot, agitated energy of the day. I even imagine long taproots, like carrots, growing down deeply into the earth to retrieve Yin for my benefit. The specific point on both feet that I use is at the beginning of the Kidney meridian, known as *Bubbling Well.* It is in the middle of the front third of the foot, just behind the ball. This breathing meditation helps me enormously when I cannot seem to calm my mind and anxiety arises. Traffic jams and post office lines are a couple of places that I regularly ground and calm myself with this technique. Another useful tool is counting your breaths while slowly breathing from the belly, not shallow chest breathing. Counting breaths replaces the mind chatter that often disturbs my falling asleep or getting back to sleep.

One of the easiest ways to nourish Yin and control Yang at bedtime is to take a mineral supplement, like Calcium and/or Magnesium. Minerals build up Yin and anchor Yang, because they are heavy. There are several shells used in Chinese herbal formulas for this purpose, including abalone shell, mother of pearl shell, oyster shell, clam shell and pearls, as well as fossilized bones. The most interesting formula that I was ever prescribed for my intractable insomnia included ground pearls and scorpions, along with lots of Yin nourishing herbs. It successfully broke the long stretch of sleepless nights I had suffered. Another strategy used in Chinese medicine for severe insomnia cases is to strongly activate the blood with herbs like Dan Shen/Red Sage Root. Similarly, regular exercise helps many people with their sleep issues.

One of the most sedative herbs for sleep and pain is Valerian root. It stinks, but is very effective. My favorite Valerian combination is by herbalist Michael Tierra, *Planetary Herbals Valerian Easy Sleep*. This balanced formula is helpful for many insomniacs. Another great sleep aid is the Chinese formula based on the Ziziphus seed/Suan Zao Ren, which nourishes the Yin and blood of the Heart and Liver. The formula is called *Suan Zao Ren Tang* and is widely available as a tablet. The single herb, Suan Zao Ren, can be toasted and ground into a powder to make tea at bedtime, or put into yogurt or pudding. It is a wonderful herb to nourish our frazzled nervous systems. Other herbs that can help sleep include Hops, Passion Flower Vine, Scullcap, Lemon Balm and Chamomile. The Hops in beer and *near beer* contributes to the sleepiness produced, but tea or capsules of Hops can be much more sedative.

And don't forget to clean up your sleep hygiene, reducing the light as bedtime approaches. Turn off the screens, wind down with calm activities, take a warm Lavender bath or foot bath.

Essential oil of Lavender or Rose Geranium can be placed on a tissue by your pillow, or applied to the inside of the wrists, to induce peaceful sleep. This is the time I also take 1 mg. Melatonin, to assure easy falling asleep. Beware, it can cause more dreams, which is disturbing for some people. An hour or so before bed is the time for your Chamomile tea or other sleep aid. Tough cases may need another dose right at bedtime. Sometimes I even have patients take a third dose of their herbs when they wake during the night.

From another point of view, sleep disorders can be a result of *adrenal exhaustion* or *adrenal burn out*. What that means is that stress has put the body into a *fight or flight* state, with the hormonal responses necessary to fight a bear, all of the time. The adrenals are one of the hormone makers that become exhausted with this endless fictional battle. They are tiny organs that sit on top of the Kidneys. The Chinese Kidney system includes the adrenals. So through Chinese medicine eyes, the adrenals will be strengthened by eating Kidney nourishing foods: anything dark in color – black, blue, purple, green. Seaweed soup is one of my favorites. Also, salty flavored foods like fish, miso and tamari, will nourish the Kidney. If *adrenal exhaustion* contributes to the insomnia, good herbs to use are Ashwaganda and Schizandra. There is a great formula by *Planetary Herbals* called *Schizandra Adrenal Complex*. In the Ayurvedic tradition of India, Ashwaganda is traditionally used as a pleasant tasting, nutritive tonic, mixed into milk. It is available in powders, pills and extracts. Ashwaganda is also used to treat anxiety. A food herb known to support the adrenals is Parsley leaf, which can be included in the diet regularly, in salads and soups.

Another sleep aid may come from supplements that affect the brain chemistry, including serotonin, which helps us sleep. Bedtime supplements for this purpose include GABA, Tryptophan and 5-HTP. And, don't take these if you are currently taking an SSRI (selective serotonin re-uptake inhibitor) anti-depressant drug or other mood changing pharmaceutical drugs, due to the possible side effect of too much serotonin (causing confusion, fever, shivering, sweating, diarrhea and muscle spasms). A carbohydrate snack in the evening would be another way to foster the production of more serotonin. Brain chemistry is very individual, so we each respond differently. If one remedy doesn't work, have hope and try another. You may just not have found your remedy yet. Julia Ross' book, *The Mood Cure*, may help you figure out which supplements are best for your needs. Another useful reference is Dr Michael Lesser's *The Brain Chemistry Diet*.

I recently heard a brilliant wellness oriented doctor from the Cleveland Clinic, Dr Michael Roizen, talk about five ways you can lower your blood pressure, in addition to a vegetable rich diet and regular exercise. He presented extensive research to back up each suggestion. These lifestyle tips seem very pertinent to our stress reduction and insomnia topic:

– Turn down the volume to 2/3 – wear ear plugs
– Forgive someone
– Get a massage
– Look at the cup half full – be hopeful
– Get more sleep

CHAPTER 6

Brain Health

LET'S FACE IT, most of us by the 50's begin to notice less mental vigor, and it seems to progress more rapidly as we age into the 60's and 70's and beyond. My father had Alzheimer's disease in his 80's, and watching his decline first hand was gruesome. Fortunately, the research into Alzheimer's is making significant inroads to understanding the progression of the disease. One of the things the research has shown is the connection between heart health and brain health, as well as, diabetes and the brain. The dietary advice is to eat a balanced healthy diet with lots of colorful fruits and vegetables; plenty of healthy fats from fish, grass fed beef, nuts and seeds, coconut, olives; and minimize sugar and refined foods to reduce inflammation, maintain level blood sugar, and improve brain and heart health.

The most cutting edge research now points to the negative impact that a high sugar, high carbohydrate, low fat diet has on the brain. The brain needs fats for fuel, not sugar. When given a high sugar, low fat diet, this can lead to high levels of insulin, creating inflammation in the brain and a reduction of mental function. The book *Grain Brain* by neurologist David Perlmutter, explores this concept, clearly showing the connection between the high carb diet and the observable injury to the brain. High blood sugar levels start a cascade of inflammation resulting in a reduction of neurotransmitters and ultimately the shrinking and stiffening of the brain. That sticky protein in wheat called gluten is one of the problems. It triggers significant inflammation, not just in the digestive systems of the sensitive, but in all of our brains. It bears doing a little experiment for a month of no sugar, no wheat to see if your mind is clearer. The wheat of today is much higher in gluten than that of the past.

Gut health = Mental Health. The healthy intestinal bacteria contribute greatly to our mental well being via the vagus nerve. A recently study with mice revealed that transplanting the gut flora from calm mice into nervous ones, made them calmer. Calm mice receiving nervous mice flora became nervous. We have know for some time that the majority of our immune responses/functions take place in the gut, but now we are seeing how much of a role that plays in mental health as well. I like to drink probiotic drinks like Kevita or miso soup for maintaining healthy intestinal flora. Yogurt, kefir, and cultured vegetables, like sauerkraut, will also replenish the gut flora. Probiotic capsules are available as well.

Do some form of healthy physical exercise 3-4 times a week. This aids with blood sugar maintenance and weight, as well as improving circulation to the brain and body.

Mental exercises like reading, puzzles, drawing, taking pictures...what ever lights up your curiosity, will keep the brain alive and functioning. Playing a musical instrument, learning a new language, anything "new" you learn helps the brain to heal. Start brushing your teeth with your non-dominant hand. In David Snowdon's book, *Aging With Grace*, he describes a group of nuns who donated their brains for the study of Alzheimer's. These women were very engaged and involved in their lives, and post mortum studies repeatedly showed degeneration in their brains, yet they were still functioning and having meaningful lives.

Social interactions are essential for brain health, connecting memories and emotions, and expanding one's world. This was another health promoting factor in Dr Snowdon's nuns' study. With the aging population, isolation is the enemy.

Herbal Aids

Turmeric has been used for 1000's of years in China and India for various ailments. The curcumin that it contains is thought to be responsible for the low rate of dementia in India, with the daily use of turmeric widespread there. I cook with turmeric regularly in curries, soups, and egg salad.

Gingko biloba is a gorgeous tree with butter yellow bi-lobed leaves in the fall. The fruit is harvested as a Kidney and brain tonic in the Chinese tradition. The leaf has been extensively researched in recent decades for its benefit on circulation to the brain and memory aid. It is usually taken as a capsule.

Bacopa benefits clear thoughts and better focus. It is available in capsules.

Holy Basil is especially useful for anxiety and restless minds. It can be used in cooking or the oil used in an atomizer. The herb is taken in capsules or teas. In India this herb is considered to be a sacred, protective plant, they call Tulsi.

Ashwaganda benefits ones vitality and will assist in regulating the sleep cycle. Poor sleep or active at night patterns ("sundowner") are often seen with dementia patients. This may help.

Sage and Rosemary can both be prepared as teas or used in cooking. Their aromatic oils are used to revive the senses and benefit the brain. Rosemary tea is used as a delightful hair rinse that invigorates the scalp. Sage tea as a rinse is good for dandruff. The scent of essential oil of rosemary is used in aromatherapy for dementia. With agitation, the scent of lavender oil is used.

Dan Shen/Red Sage root is a special variety of sage from China with potent healing properties for the brain, the heart and the liver. It is used to invigorate circulation and nourish the blood, while also calming the emotions and reducing inflammation. It is used in formulas by a trained herbal practitioner.

Prevagen is a supplement based on a jellyfish protein that illuminates in the dark. This protein reduces a mineral build up in the brain, allowing for more clarity in memory and thoughts. It really helped me last year when I feared that my mind was going. Remembering Latin names of plants, which used to be easy for me, became a struggle. Prevagen made a huge difference for me. It also helped my sleep. It is available in your local pharmacy.

We have the power to change the course of mental decline if we stay vigilant to nourish and protect our beautiful brains. I learned recently that the brain has 100,000 miles of blood vessels. Keep it flowing!

References:

Grain Brain by David Perlmutter, MD. The surprising truth about wheat, carbs and sugar - your brain's silent killers.

Wheat Belly Cookbook by William Davis, MD. No wheat, no sugar, yummy recipes.

Aging with Grace by David Snowdon, PhD. The beautiful story of the nuns' brain study.

III.

Fall

Have a sense of gratitude to everything, even difficult emotions, because of their potential to wake you up. - Pema Chodron

CHAPTER 1

Gratitude Heals the Mind and Body

MY FAVORITE HOLIDAY of the year comes at the end of November...Thanksgiving. Imagine a whole day dedicated to being thankful! When that attitude of gratitude is practiced regularly, it can have far reaching benefits to both physical and mental health, changing our world view from glass half empty to glass half full, just by a shift in perception.

Research studies at the University of California at Davis, led by Robert Emmons, have shown the wide reaching benefits of practicing gratitude, including better sleep, improved heart health with protection from heart attacks, fewer illness symptoms, stronger immunity, and a more optimistic outlook about the future. Grateful people take better care of themselves in general, and engage in more health protective behaviors, including more exercise, better diets and better stress management. Emmons' studies have shown that those practicing gratitude regularly experience higher levels of positive emotions such as joy, enthusiasm, love, happiness and optimism. Additionally, the practice of gratitude as a discipline protects a person from the destructive impulses of envy, resentment, greed and bitterness. Even spending just a few minutes daily in a state of gratitude can be transformational, helping us to replace fear, anxiety and worry with joy, happiness and peace, resulting in a more balanced body and mind.

An interesting survey was conducted by psychologist Christopher Peterson, from the University of Michigan, of more than 3000 Americans after the tragedy on 9/11/2001. The survey showed that in the face of adversity, there was a surge in feelings of gratitude. It was concluded that gratitude in the aftermath of tragedy can help buffer people from the negative effects of stress, making them less like to suffer from post-traumatic stress disorder. Cultivate gratitude!

One of the easiest and most effective ways to cultivate a grateful attitude is to begin keeping a gratitude journal, taking a few minutes to acknowledge 3-5 things that you feel grateful for each day. Another tool is to write a letter of gratitude to someone who you care about. It also helps to surround yourself with others who have a similarly grateful attitude, and limit your contact with pessimistic friends.

Dr Andrew Weil says in his new book, *Spontaneous Happiness*: "From the research data that I have reviewed, I consider expressing gratitude to be one of the very best strategies to enhance emotional well being, right up there with fish oil, physical activity, and managing negative thoughts."

So much stress and bad moods occur during this time of year between Halloween and the beginning of the New Year. Energetically, this is the time to be quiet, inward and contemplative, so that we may restore our reserves. Instead, we find ourselves overly busy, shopping like maniacs, exposed to a highly commercial world and partying like twenty year olds. Perhaps this year if we can cultivate gratitude, it will help us to endure the holiday stresses with more joy and peace.

The English poet William Blake said it best: "The thankful receiver bears a plentiful harvest." Happy Thanks Giving!

For more information on "gratitude therapies" refer to:

— *Spontaneous Happiness* by Andrew Weil, MD (2011)

— *Thanks!: How the New Science of Gratitude Can Make You Happier* by Robert Emmons (2007)

— *The Gratitude Effect* by Dr John Demartini (2008)

— www.spiritualityandpractice.com/practices/practices.php?id=11

— Gratefulness.org

CHAPTER 2

Breast Health

October is "Breast Cancer Awareness Month." Traditional Chinese Medicine (TCM) would suggest that energizing and nourishing the Liver promotes healthy breasts. TCM describes the body's energy as Qi, which circulates throughout the body in pathways, carrying both blood and nutrients to all parts. Cancer is viewed as an extreme case of stagnation of the Qi, blood and fluids. The Liver has an instrumental role in the healthy movement of Qi, blood and fluids. The breasts and genitals are areas that the flow of Liver Qi can easily become stagnant.

Tips to keep the Liver pathways open and smoothly flowing: Regular exercise; Wholesome, fiber-rich foods; Kind thoughts for yourself and others; Forgiveness. Our society is suffering with a bad case of toxic Liver Qi stagnation, witnessed in the widespread lack of civility and tone of cruelty that exists today.

Food wise, the Liver benefits from fruits and vegetables (especially the green ones), whole grains and beans, and clean animal products. The burdens that we place on the Liver come mostly with bad choices: greasy, fried foods; sugar and other refined foods; artificially flavored, sweetened and colored "pseudo-foods"; and hateful thoughts. These all can cause a sluggish Liver, which leads to a variety of ailments including painful breasts, mood swings, irritability, depression, anxiety, eye disorders, painful menses and poor digestion.

Dr Andrew Weil's newsletter suggested that "one of the best defenses against breast cancer may well be diet. A growing and impressive body of research reveals that what you eat and drink can help protect you from the disease."

He goes on to suggest that women should regularly eat the following:

– Whole, non-GMO soy foods like edamame, tofu, tempeh and soy milk (check with your doctor if you can have soy)*
– Fruits and vegetables – at least 9 daily servings (especially bright colors)
– Green tea – at least 1 cup, or up to 5 cups daily
– Fish – aim for 2 or 3 servings per week of oily fish such as salmon or cod
– Flax seeds - sprinkle 2 Tablespoons of ground seeds on food daily

Dr. Weil's "Foods to Limit or Avoid" include: sugar, red meat, charred meats, partially hydrogenated oils, and alcohol.

TCM would also use breathing or stretching exercises that have a calming effect on the mind. A peaceful mind will greatly enhance Liver health, and, in turn, breast health. Relax and breathe in peace and calmness; then, exhale all of the stress, negative thoughts and feelings stuck inside. A few rounds of "in with peace, out with stress" and the world is a prettier place, or at least your Liver thinks so. One of the best resources I have seen for further instruction is *Better Breast Health Naturally with Chinese Medicine* by Honora Lee Wolfe and Bob Flaws (Blue Poppy Press). They propose that breast health, whether you are dealing with benign cysts, pre-period tenderness, or more serious masses, all comes down to regulating the smooth flow of Liver Qi. Start now, and hopefully, you can avoid a whole range of troubles. The best foods for preventing and treating cancer will follow.

Anti-Cancer Foods

Foods High In Beta Carotene
This includes yellow and orange vegetables like carrots, yams and pumpkin.

Cruciferous Vegetables

This family includes cabbage, kale, collards, broccoli, Brussels sprouts, cauliflower, turnips, radishes, mustard greens. In their raw form, these can inhibit thyroid function so mostly have them cooked.

Dark Leafy Greens

These are rich in minerals, chlorophyll and other cancer fighting anti-oxidants. Include romaine, endive, spinach, dandelion greens, arugula, watercress. All types of seaweeds, such as wakame, kombu, hiziki, arame, nori, dulse, etc.

Onion Family of Vegetables

This includes onions, garlic, leeks, chives, scallions and shallots. They all contain anti-cancer sulfur compounds.

Medicinal Mushrooms

These foods are used to boost the immune system and have potent anti-cancer properties. The best ones to use as food are shitake, maitake, and enoki. Others may be used in supplements as capsules, tinctures, or teas. These may include ganoderma (reishi), cordyceps, wood ears, polyporus and chaga. (www.mitobi.com)

Colorful Fruits

Apples, grapes, apricots, peaches and berries all have powerful anti-cancer properties. Citrus peels are made into teas to benefit digestion.

Whole Grains And Beans

Brown rice, barley, quinoa, oats and millet are all good choices. Fermented soybean (miso and tempeh), edamame, tofu and soymilk are good proteins, as are lima beans, mung beans, and garbanzo beans. Beans help reduce toxicity.

High Quality Proteins

Low fat yogurt, fish and beans are the best protein sources. Choose fish that are low in pollutants and environmentally friendly. Wild salmon is rich in Omega 3 oils. For lists of healthy fish: seafoodwatch.org (Monterey Bay Aquarium).

Healing Beverages

Vegetable juice, green tea, ginger tea, roasted chicory or dandelion root tea, holy basil (tulsi) tea, lemon juice in water, citrus peel tea

Best To Avoid The Following: The 3 refined "whites": sugar, flour and salt; processed foods filled with chemical additives and preservatives; poor quality oils and fats, hydrogenated oils, deep fried foods, high fat foods; alcohol

CHAPTER 3

Indian Summer is Here

THESE LONG, HOT, last days of summer comprise a fifth season of the year, Indian Summer or Late Summer. According to Traditional Chinese Medicine (TCM), this season is associated with the Earth Element and the organs of digestion: Stomach, Spleen and Pancreas. The best strategy for harmony with the season and support of the digestive system, will be to choose easily digested, simple meals of fruits, vegetables, complex carbohydrates like brown rice, quinoa, oats, beans, root vegetables, and proteins like chicken or fish. The full-sweet flavor is the one that most nourishes us. Unfortunately, our taste buds have been hijacked to believe that empty sweets also count as food. Not true. Actually, too much sugar ingestion contributes to multiple vitamin and mineral deficiencies. I recently learned that the average American consumes 130 pounds of sugar per year...that is one-third of a pound per day! Refined sugar is addictive and not a good substitute for wholesome, full-sweet flavored foods like carrots, oatmeal, and apples. So we need to be careful not to fall into the quicksand pit of sugar, especially now. Instead, choose a variety of full-sweet flavored, nutrient dense foods. The digestive system is a major source of vitality. Poor digestion contributes to low energy, weak immunity and phlegm/fluid accumulations. When our digestive systems are strong, we are better able to digest ideas and information. TCM teaches us that mindful eating promotes good digestion. Chewing well. Not distracted by driving, watching TV, etc, while we eat.

In her lovely herbal, *Healing with the Herbs of Life*, Lesley Tierra says: *The quality of late summer is transformation, symbolic of digestive functions and our shift from warming spring and summer to cooling fall and winter...its a time of stability and rootedness, qualities that nourish and balance so we withstand the changes of upcoming fall.* In preparation for the fall that is just around the corner, we now begin to reduce the raw foods, icy drinks and juices.

Some of my favorite herb teas to benefit the digestion are the seeds that we use in cooking - cardamon, caraway, fennel, anise, coriander, cumin – these can be made into teas by simply steeping a round teaspoon of the crushed seeds in boiling water for 10 minutes. Strain and drink daily. Ginger tea is another important staple for the digestion. Cut several slices of the fresh root and lightly simmer for 5-10 minutes. Recently I discovered ginger juice in a bottle *(The Ginger People* brand*)*, a quick alternative to the above.

Hawthorn berries are another great digestive. The variety that grows in the US is especially good for the heart while the Chinese variety is better for digestion, especially of fatty, greasy foods and animal products. In a large Asian market you will find this herb in many forms. One of them is a simple candy called *Haw Flakes.* Hawthorn is also an ingredient in two very valuable digestive aids, *Curing Pill* and *Bao He Wan. Curing Pill (Kang Ning Wan)* is effective for many types of upset stomach, indigestion, nausea and diarrhea. It can be very helpful for those with a sensitive digestive system. The other brilliant digestive, *Preserve Harmony Pill (Bao He Wan)*, would be used in cases of indigestion, primarily due to overeating, in which there is belching, heartburn, constipation or diarrhea. Another important Earth remedy is *Six Gentlemen Pill (Liu Jun Zi Wan)* which enhances and regulates digestion, strengthens immunity and vitality, and transforms phlegm. This is for the person who is tired and weak with a pale, swollen tongue, and poor digestion. Simple meals. No extremes. Mindful eating. These are our keys to balance and harmony in this Earth season that is upon us.

CHAPTER 4

Lung Health in Autumn

AUTUMN ARRIVES WITH cold nights, shorter days, colorful leaves and the beginning of cold and flu season. The Lungs and Large Intestines are the organ systems that are prominent during autumn, leading to an increased vulnerability in the respiratory system. There are many natural remedies we can employ to keep our lungs healthy in the months to come, as well as treat them in the event sickness befalls us.

First, breathe...deeply, slowly, regularly. The lungs take energy from the air we breathe. If you are sitting hunched over a computer or a desk all day, the lungs cannot receive much volume of air, so take breaks to expand the chest and breathe. Recently, a patient told me that she was falling down easily and felt that she was not very well connected to the earth. I gave her a breathing exercise to imagine that carrot-like roots were growing out of the bottoms of her feet and going deep into the earth to ground and balance her. This exercise can also be useful when we get "too much in our heads" and cannot turn off the endless rambling of the mind. Stop and breathe...deeply, slowly, regularly, through your feet. This helps us deal with pain, physical or emotional, as well as anxiety, fear and panic. And, deep breathing heals the lungs.

When dealing with lung issues, a diet to support them is essential. Foods that are especially useful are carrots, beets, sweet potatoes, pears, almonds, rice, barley, oats, white colored beans, mushrooms and fish. One of the best herbs to strengthen the lungs and the immune system is Astragalus. It can be taken as a supplement or cooked into soups. The medicinal mushrooms, such as shitake and maitake, are very useful to boost immunity during this time of year, and can be cooked with eggs, vegetables and grains. Make sure that the bowels are moving regularly. This will benefit the lungs since these two organs work closely together. Flax seeds, olive oil, sesame seeds, walnuts, and plenty of fruits and vegetables will all promote healthy bowel movements.

When addressing lung and sinus conditions, one of the first things to observe is whether it is acute (sudden onset) or chronic (lasting many weeks, months or years). If an acute cough is accompanied by chills, fever, body ache, headache, sneezing, sore throat and/or runny nose, a Chinese doctor would tell you that you have been "invaded by wind" or caught a viral infection. In the early stages when chills are prominent, fresh Ginger tea is the best medicine. Grate about a thumb size piece and simmer for 5-10 minutes with a pint of water. Drink several cups of this throughout the day and bundle up. As you sweat, the wind (virus) will be released and you will feel better. Warm salt water gargles will ease sore throat. Ginger tea will also be the best medicine if the condition includes nausea or vomiting. If fever predominates, strong peppermint tea is the best medicine. Use 2 or 3 bags per cup and drink several cups throughout the day. If you have access to Chinese medicines, Yin Qiao pills works great. Soups and light foods are the best nutrition for all types of acute coughs and colds. Season foods with thyme, sage or oregano, all of which treat a variety of lung infections.

For chronic coughs, as well as acute ones that are not related to sudden viral infections, it is necessary to observe the associated phlegm (or no phlegm). If there is no phlegm or it is a very dry cough, hot water with the addition of honey and lemon juice will be soothing. Also moistening would be fruits, soy foods, almonds, oily fish (like salmon), and teas made from Slippery Elm, Marshmallow or Licorice root.

If the phlegm is yellow, that shows heat/inflammation in the lungs. The darker yellow, brown, green phlegm may signify a bacterial infection. If there is a significant fever, do not delay being seen by your doctor. Some of the herbs used for this type of lung condition could include Echinacea, Golden Seal, Mullein or Honeysuckle tea. If you have access to a Chinatown, my favorite remedy is a pill called Qing Qi Hua Tan Wan. Healing foods would include seaweed soup, daikon radish, bitter greens, celery, pears, apples and basmati rice, while avoiding spicy foods and alcohol.

If the cough includes white or clear, frothy, copious phlegm, this shows that the lungs have an accumulation of dampness and/or cold. This is the time for a spicy soup with plenty of ginger, peppers, garlic and onions, and stay away from all foods that you observe create more phlegm, such as salads, dairy products, sweets, and fried foods. Tea made from Sage or Thyme will aid the expectoration of the phlegm. Use 1 teaspoon per cup of boiling water and steep for 10 minutes.

There are several cough syrups that are available at natural food stores. My all around favorite is Planetary Herbal's Old Indian Wild Cherry Syrup. It can be used for a variety of coughs. My favorite dry cough syrups are Han's Honey Loquat Syrup and Fritillary-Loquat Cough Syrup.

The sinuses are an extension of the Lung organ system. If they are congested, using either a few drops of Eucalyptus, Peppermint or Lavender oil in a steamer can open the nasal passages. If the sinus problem becomes an infection with yellow or green discharge, that is the time for Golden Seal, Honeysuckle, or the Chinese pill, Bi Yan Pian.

Keeping the lungs healthy in autumn may also include more expressions of sadness and grief, the emotions housed by the lungs. So don't dismay if you are feeling blue lately…it is part of being in tune with the autumn season. This too will pass.

CHAPTER 5

Menopause and Other Middle Age Stresses

MY LAST PERIOD came the day after I turned 56. For women around the world, average age is 51. The time leading up to the cessation of menstruation is called peri-menopause, and can last several years or more, with all sorts of irregularities. Menopause is officially here when you have not had a menstrual period for one year. Many women choose the hormone replacement (HRT) route when the symptoms are severe, but there are some serious possible side effects. The real dangers with HRT occur when used long term (more than 5 years) and in high doses. Personally, I had strokes, breast and uterine cancers in my family history, so HRT was never a safe choice.

The other danger with HRT, in my opinion, can be associated with the denial of the aging process, using hormones as a "fountain of youth." The current craze (at least in California) is "bio-identical hormones" which logically sound safer than synthetic ones, but there are no long term studies done with them to actually confirm safety. I do, however, believe that bio-identical hormones are a better choice, for me, if absolutely necessary. Much of the discomforts of menopause can be lessened greatly with herbs and nutrition. Menopause is NOT a disease, it is a life transition.

In her books, Christiane Northrop, MD, brilliantly discusses this time as "a mind-body revolution that brings the greatest opportunity for growth since adolescence." She also advises that peri-menopausal and menopausal women will control their weight more easily if they avoid refined grains, and limit grains in general. Laurie Steelsmith, naturopathic doctor, acupuncturist and practitioner of Chinese medicine, has written a great manual for women's health. In it she describes menopause "not as a loss of youth but as a time of great potential and joy." She quotes Dr Bob Flaws' description of menopause as the time a woman becomes "the mother of her community and a fountain of wisdom."

As the estrogen production by the ovaries begins to wane, the adrenals take over, making the decline in estrogen less dramatic. However, by the time many women are in their 40's, life's stresses have significantly depleted their adrenals, so they are not able to help ease the transition into menopause. The adrenal glands sit on top of our kidneys, in the low back, and produce cortisol, the "fight or flight" hormone. This peaks when our life is threatened and we must flee. Unfortunately, many of us are now hormonally fighting a ferocious lion all of the time. Over time, the adrenals become exhausted and are unable to function normally, leaving us feeling in a constant state of overload...tired, but wired. Vitamins B and C are depleted with stress. One of the worst things for the adrenals is drinking excessive amounts of coffee, like beating the dead horse to do more. I wonder how much of the hormone hype being pitched to men about "low testosterone" would be more correctly diagnosed as adrenal exhaustion.

Some of the herbs that are considered to be restorative to the adrenals and nervous system include: Lemon Balm, Nettle leaf, Licorice root (not with hypertension or edema), Parsley, Oats, Scullcap and Passion Flower vine. Seaweed, oily fish like salmon (or fish oil capsules), and dark colored-mineral rich foods, will also support the adrenals and kidneys. With severe menopausal symptoms or severe stress, it may be best to seek out a professional herbalist or naturopath in your area to make a custom formula for you.

That said, there are a few over the counter herbs and supplements that may be helpful for the 3 most annoying symptoms of menopause: hot flashes, vaginal dryness and emotional instability. A black cohosh product from Europe called *Remifemin* is fabulous for hot flashes. It is a mint flavored tablet you chew up 1-2 times a day. Within a short time, the hot flashes are reduced in the majority of women. Chinese medicine would use one of several formulas containing a black herb called Rehmannia root. *Zhi Bai Di Huang Wan (Rehmannia 6 Herbs Pill*

Modified) is used for hot flashes. Mint tea, celery, cucumbers, mung beans and soy foods, may also help clear the fire. Vitamin E helps lubricate dryness when taken internally. Eating healthy fats like nuts, seeds, avocados, olive oil, coconut oil, and fish, will also help. At the same time avoid the most drying agents – coffee, alcohol and hot spicy foods.

The emotions are the most challenging to treat, and probably need individual treatment. I do, however, like using a couple of Chinese formulas for this that are pretty easy to find in pill form. *Suan Zao Ren Tang (Ziziphus Seed Decoction)* nourishes the Heart and Liver and helps with insomnia. *Jia Wei Xiao Yao Wan (Relaxed Wander)* regulates the Liver and strengthens the digestion, especially suited to the roller coaster type of emotions. If there is a history of very heavy periods or anemia, *Gui Pi Tang (Restore the Spleen Decoction)* may be indicated. Calcium and magnesium supplements may also fortify the nervous system and improve sleep, especially taken at bedtime.

Traditional Chinese Medicine looks at menopause as a time when there is a decline in an aspect of the Kidney energy called Kidney Jing (or Essence). It is the genetic material we inherit from mom and dad, like a trust fund. How well (or not) we managed our lifestyle choices, stresses, and diet, determines the amount of Jing we have left by the time peri-menopause occurs. One of my mentors was once asked by a young student when the best time was to prepare for menopause. His answer was, "In your 20's." Translation: Don't waste that Jing trust fund in youth. Kidney Jing can be supported by eating the following foods: mussels, oysters, anchovy, clams, chicken, fertile eggs, spirulina and chlorella powders, dairy products (from cows, goats or sheep), royal jelly (from bees), Lycii berries, and black sesame seeds. And, most important of all is moderation in all aspects of life to preserve what Jing remains in the trust fund.

References:

The Wisdom of Menopause by Dr Christiane Northrop – she takes a wholistic approach with all of the details from western medicine presented clearly. A must have book for aging sisters.

The Secret Pleasures of Menopause by Dr Christiane Northrop – she takes the inspiring premise that Menopause is the beginning of life, not the end, especially with our sexuality.

Natural Choices for Women's Health by Dr Laurie Steelsmith – a fabulous health manual that unites Eastern and Western thoughts on women's conditions. Excellent reference.

Herbal Healing for Women by Rosemary Gladstar – she is a pioneer in the herb world.

Women's Herbs, Women's Health by Christopher Hobbs and Kathi Keville – two more pioneers with great herb advice.

CHAPTER 6

Sex and the Aging Woman

I HAVE HAD many decades of incredible, loving sex. At 63, unpartnered, sex has moved to the back of my mind. I have not tested the waters for a while, but have lots of aging married women as patients and friends who share their bedroom stories with me. The most disturbing to hear is the obligatory painful sex, often performed with their Viagra fueled husbands. The invention of Viagra-type drugs was generally not so good for many older women, while being a big boon for aging male sexuality. For women there has never really been an effective sex organ drug. Our most important sex organ is our brain. Therein lies the key to good sex as we age. Each of us has our unique sexual thoughts that can trigger ecstasy. Memories are often the food for such thoughts. Fortunately, I still have a great memory bank. Talk to your partner.

One of my friends reminded me that the skin is also a primary sex organ. Everyone can benefit from touch therapy. Even if intercourse is not an option or choice, there are so many ways to experience pleasurable touch. Intimacy can be shared in a myriad of ways. The World Health Organization defines sexual health as ...*a state of physical, emotional, mental and social well-being in relation to sexuality; it is not merely the absence of disease, dysfunction or infirmity. Sexual health requires a positive and respectful approach to sexuality and sexual relationships, as well as the possibility of having pleasurable and safe sexual experiences, free of coercion, discrimination and violence.*

Now, what can be done about that painful sex? One of the most common causes is *vaginal atrophy*. The tissues of the vulva and vagina are kept moist and supple by estrogen. At menopause the ovaries stop making estrogen. The adrenals and adipose tissue continue to be a small source, but some women may need to supplement with hormones. With fears abundant in the use of oral hormone replacement therapy, one safer option is to use a topical estrogen cream on the genitals. This can be sufficient to reduce the sand paper feeling that intercourse can cause. In severe cases, systemic hormones may be indicated. Bio-identical hormones may be safer, but there are no long term studies to substantiate that as truth. Lack of interest for women may suggest a DHEA, testosterone, or thyroid hormone deficiency. Your doctor can order a hormone panel to see exactly what is off with your hormones. Long term use of hormone replacement therapy can be risky. Menopause is NOT a deficiency of estrogen. It is a natural part of our life cycle.

My mother was put on Premarin at age 40 when she had a hysterectomy because of cervical cancer. She stayed on that estrogen drug (made from pregnant mare's urine and initially thought to be a fountain of youth) until after having a mastectomy for breast cancer at 65. Lung cancer finally killed her at 79. When I learned that like the breasts, the lungs also have estrogen receptors, I saw the connection. I believe that her 2nd and 3rd cancers were caused by being on Premarin for 25 years. Hormone replacement therapy is a serious choice, so be sure to look at all of your options and risks.

Chinese medicine works extremely well to treat peri-menopausal symptoms. One of the remedies that was very helpful for my hot flashes and night sweats was a product made from Black Cohosh root, called *Remifemin*. A trained herbalist can help you find solutions. From the point of view of Chinese medicine, the herbal focus is on restoring Kidney Essence and Liver Blood, while limiting the inflaming foods. This is a great time to learn about meditation and breathing exercises to stay calm, as the flames of menopause flare. Some of the foods recommended for Kidney Essence are wheat germ, mussels, oysters and fertile eggs. To nourish the Blood, go for anything green. The chlorophyll molecule responsible for that green color is almost identical to the hemoglobin molecule in red blood cells, so it is an easy conversion for the body to do.

Aromatherapist Peter Holmes, sells an incredible topical vaginal serum, *Triple Goddess Rose Oil,* made from hazelnut oil and organic Damask Rose oil (snowlotus.org). It was developed by herbalist and acupuncturist, Rachel Koenig, for her patients. The product is beneficial for the thinning or dry vaginal tissue. The incredible scent of roses promotes joy, and is healing to the reproductive organs. It can be used as a lubricant as well as for improving libido. The hazelnut oil has a compatible pH for the delicate vaginal tissue. I started using it in the making of my lip balms and find that hazelnut is the perfect oil for the upstairs lips too.

Herbalist, Rosemary Gladstar, suggests the following topical treatments for vaginal atrophy and thinning vaginal tissue: Aloe Vera gel + Slippery Elm powder. Mix the powder into the gel to make a paste which will soothe and lubricate inflamed, dry tissue. This paste can also be used as a sexual lubricant. Rosemary also suggests using herbal salves made with Comfrey + Aloe or Calendula + Comfrey + St John's wort. *Avena Botanicals* sells a product with those herbs plus Olive oil and Clary Sage essential oil, called *Vaginal Dryness Oil*. Herbalists Christopher Hobbs and Kathi Keville suggest the following topical treatment: 2 oz. Almond oil + 6 drops Rose Geranium essential oil, 6 drops Lavender essential oil, 1 drop Neroli oil (optional) and vitamin E oil capsules, totaling about 1500 IU, opened. They call this remedy *Rejuvenation Oil*, with instructions to apply to labia or vagina as needed.

Kegel exercises (repetitions of tightening and relaxing the muscles on the pelvic floor) may promote better genital circulation as well as lubrication. Internally staying hydrated and supplementing with vitamin E and Omega 3 fatty acids from flax, fish, and evening primrose, may also be helpful in staying juicy. Royal jelly, manufactured by the bees, is another internal remedy for more supple genitals, which nourishes the Kidney Essence.

Good circulation is an important part of healthy sexual responses, not just to produce a male erection, but also for women's arousal. The herb Ginkgo Biloba leaf has shown some benefit for sexual dysfunction, male and female, caused as a side effect to anti-depressant medications. This herb was first popularized as an aid to better brain and heart health by improving blood flow. Exercise is essential for healthy circulation. Most people feel more sexy when they are getting regular exercise.

Living life with passion is a worthy goal at any age. Lust for life fosters curiosity and fascination with each day. If sex is not that interesting, look further to see if passion is lacking elsewhere in your life. Do what you love to do and when your cup is full, let it spill over on your beloved, in bed and otherwise. How about starting with exchanging foot massages, my favorite foreplay.

References:

www.who.int/reproductivehealth/topics/sexual_health/sh_definitions/en/
Mating in Captivity: Unlocking Erotic Intelligence by Dr Esther Perel
The Secret Pleasures of Menopause by Dr Christian Northrup
Sex and the Seasoned Woman by Gail Sheehy
Women's Herbs, Women's Health by Christopher Hobbs, LAc and Kathi Keville
The Family Herbal by Rosemary Gladstar

IV.

Winter

Look at a tree, a flower, a plant. Let your awareness rest upon it.
How still they are, how deeply rooted in being.
Allow Nature to teach you stillness. - Eckhart Tolle

CHAPTER 1

Dying at the New Year: Year of the Earth Rat

LIFE GAVE ME a precious New Year's gift today: The most critically ill patient I have ever worked with, the most severe physical suffering I have ever tried to relieve. And, the most caring, loving, devoted wife attending to his needs. Her loving kindness profoundly touched my heart. This gift came to shake me out of my self-pity for the extra twenty pounds I am carrying. I wasn't going to go to the Ni family's New Year's party Sunday because I felt too fat to be seen. How much easier it is to have compassion for the suffering of others than it is to feel compassion for oneself. I must learn to love myself and attend to my vulnerabilities as tenderly as I watched Pam today care for Myles. She showed me true love, the nitty gritty, painful part of love – watching your beloved dying.

Myles looked a lot like the man in the movie, *The Diving Bell and the Butterfly*, though with much less mental acuity. His dementia was severe, but there was still a sparkle in the one eye he could see out of. He even smiled when I told him goodbye. His broken body is gnarled by stokes, arthritis, extreme foot and leg ulcers, and he screams with pain, but when Pam asked him if he wanted to die, he emphatically said "NO!" I don't know if I can really do anything for Myles' body and mind, but I know that I can do a lot for his wife with my support and kindness. As I helped her dress his ulcers with Manuka honey, it nearly took my breath away, but Pam didn't flinch. Her love never wavered for a second.

May we all be so fortunate to have an angel to love us like this at the end. How shallow I feel for whining about my adipose and almost missing my favorite celebration of the year.

CHAPTER 2

February: Heart Health Awareness Month

FEBRUARY WAS PROCLAIMED to be American Heart Month in 1963 in an attempt to raise public awareness of heart disease, the number one killer of both men and women in the United States. One in every three deaths here is from heart disease and strokes, equal to 2,200 deaths per day. Those at greater risk include women 55 or older; men 45 or older; and anyone with a family history of early heart disease. We have the power to prevent much of heart disease with diet, lifestyle and attitude changes.

One of the missions of the American Heart Association has been to educate Americans about how to have healthy hearts (http://www.heart.org/HEARTORG/). In the US, the most common type of heart disease is coronary artery disease, which can lead to a heart attack when the arteries that feed the heart muscle become blocked. For men, heart attack symptoms often include severe chest pain that may radiate down the left arm, the sensation that an elephant is sitting on his chest, and shortness of breath. Women's heart attack symptoms are often mistaken for something else: pain in the stomach, chest, arm, jaw, neck, and/or back (maybe not as severe as for a man); indigestion, nausea or heart burn; extreme and unexplainable fatigue; shortness of breath; anxiety or sleep disturbances; and cold sweats. Unfortunately, many women die from their first heart attack, missing these warning signs.

So how do we prevent heart disease? The American Heart Association's guidelines are:

1) Watch your weight.

2) Quit smoking and stay away from second hand smoke.

3) Control your cholesterol and blood pressure.

4) If you drink alcohol, drink only in moderation.

5) Get active and eat healthy.

6) Talk to your doctor about taking aspirin every day if you are a man over the age of 45 or a woman over 55.

7) Manage stress.

One of the most reliable markers for predicting heart disease is a measure of general inflammation in the body, CRP (C - Reactive Protein). If your number is under 1, you are doing great; between 1 and 2 shows average amounts of inflammation; over 3 indicates high levels of inflammation and high risk of developing many diseases, including heart disease. This is an easy piece of information to gain from a simple blood test. The Mediterranean Diet, which includes abundant fruits and vegetables, whole grains and beans, nuts and seeds, fish and olive oil, is very effective in reducing inflammation. (See my next article on "Inflammation" for more details.)

Know your numbers…it gives you the power to see inside your body and make changes to improve your health. Other valuable numbers to know include the following:

1) **BMI (Body Mass Index)** – is one of the indicators of body fat, calculated by dividing your weight (in kilograms) by the square of your height (in meters). Ideal is 25 or below; 26-30 is overweight; and above 30 is obese.

2) **Waist Size** – this measures the amount of "belly fat" which can contribute to heart disease and diabetes. Ideal waist size is less than ½ of your height. Stress creates the hormone cortisol which leads to belly fat. Reducing stress is of paramount importance.

3) **Blood Sugar** – elevated blood sugar leads to diabetes and heart disease. Fasting blood sugar should be below 100.

4) **Blood Pressure** – is an important indicator of heart health. 120/80 is ideal. Over 140/90 is considered to be hypertension.

5) **Cholesterol** – several measurements are used: LDL ("bad" cholesterol), HDL ("good" cholesterol); overall cholesterol level. LDL should be below 100; HDL should be above 40 for men and 55 for women (the higher the better); overall cholesterol should be below 200. TRIGLYCERIDES are another important blood fat to keep track of, keeping this number below 150. Triglycerides go up with too many sweets, refined carbohydrates and alcohol.

When it comes to eating a heart healthy diet the following guidelines may be helpful:

1) Eat plenty of fruits and vegetables, whole grains and beans. These are all rich in fiber which helps to reduce inflammation and lower cholesterol.

2) Eat fish several times a week. The Omega 3 oils that they contain greatly benefit the heart. This is particularly useful for reducing elevated triglycerides.

3) Choose lean meats and poultry. The fatty meats are high in saturated fats which can lead to heart disease. Choose low fat dairy products as well. Free range, fertile eggs contain less saturated fat and cholesterol than factory farmed eggs.

4) Avoid trans fats (hydrogenated oils). These are not digestible and contribute to many diseases.

5) Limit refined white flour and sugar. Both of these can cause inflammation.

6) Limit salt intake. Excessive consumption of salt can raise blood pressure.

7) Dark chocolate is a heart healthy sweet treat due to its flavonols, also contained in apples, cranberries, red wine, onions and tea.

8) According to Traditional Chinese Medicine, some of the most beneficial foods for heart health would include:

Celery, mushrooms, tomatoes, bananas, corn silk tea – lower blood pressure.

Apples, asparagus, oats, rye, amaranth, beans, hawthorn berries, green tea – reduce cholesterol

Cherries, berries, red grapes, pomegranates, beets, carrots, greens – nourish the blood and strengthen the heart.

Black wood ear (mu er) and shitake mushrooms, turmeric, ginger, onions, garlic, seaweed – move blood, reduce stagnation, improve heart health.

Last but far from least, is a cheerful mental attitude to keep the heart healthy. In 2010 a 10 year study showed that those who demonstrated positive emotions had a 22% lower risk of developing heart disease. If this area is a challenge for you, might I suggest meditation, exercise, remembering gratitude or watching comedies that make you laugh.

Happy heart healthy Valentine's Day!

CHAPTER 3

Inflammation: Causes and Cures

ONE OF THE biggest predictors of how well we age is the amount of inflammation present in our bodies. The major killer diseases, such as cancer, heart disease, and Alzheimer's, as well as the discomforts of gastritis, arthritis, gingivitis, and the many other –itises, all begin with inflammation. When an organ is inflamed, disease follows. Over time that fire in the tissues or cells can become life threatening. Some of the best cures to reduce inflammation are found in colorful fruits and vegetables. The other vital component to fire reduction is to avoid unhealthy fats, denatured grains, refined sugars, and foods heavy laden in artificial flavorings, colorings and preservatives.

In recent years the medical world has awakened to the huge connection between diet and health. One of the measurable factors that your doctor may use to determine disease risks is your level of CRP (C-Reactive Proteins) in the blood. It is now know that this is a more reliable pointer to the possibility of heart disease than merely looking at cholesterol levels. It will also show the amount of inflammation generally present in the body.

Dr Andrew Weil, a brilliant Harvard trained doctor, has created an "Anti-Inflammatory Diet & Pyramid" as a "blueprint for a lifetime of optimum nutrition" (go to drweil.com for the details). My article "Eating a Rainbow" outlines many of the beneficial fruits and vegetables that he suggests.

Now for the trouble makers that we all need to limit, or better yet, avoid:

Unhealthy Fats: The worst of these are the trans-fats, or hydrogenated oils. These are huge contributors to inflammation and a host of diseases, including cancer and heart disease. Saturated fats, which mostly originate from animals, create inflammation. Instead, use oils such as olive oil and sesame oil and include fresh nuts and seeds for their range of healthy polyunsaturated and monounsaturated oils. Flax seeds, pumpkin seeds, chia seeds, and oily fish like salmon and sardines, are all high in the healthy Omega 3 oils which reduce inflammation throughout the body and boost our immunity.

Denatured Grains: Refined wheat berries are stripped of all their healthy bran, fiber and nutrients, and what is left is a white sticky substance that is formed into bread, cookies and cakes. When I was a kid in elementary school, we made glue for crafts from white flour and water. Sound familiar? In our bodies this gummy substance contributes to inflammation due to its lack of fiber to move it through. Strive to make at least half of your grain products whole and unrefined, such as whole wheat bread, rye bread, whole grain pasta, steel cut oats, and brown rice.

Refined Sugars: Let's be honest...sugar is a drug! Most of us are hooked and it is a tough addiction to face down. I know this first hand having grown up on unlimited amounts; as a 60 year old, my inner sugar addict kid still associates sweets with pleasure and comfort. We all know the damage that sugar can do to the teeth over time, but the more serious problem is the amount of inflammation that it creates. Cancer cells thrive in a high sugar environment. The problem is not the unrefined sugar in carrots, beets and cherries, but rather the refined, high calorie-no nutrient, white crystalline substance that causes the trouble. It often takes some training to even recognize the mild sweet flavor in brown rice, chicken and squash.

Artifical Chemical Additives: Our liver and kidneys are responsible for protecting us from dangerous chemicals, both endogenous and exogenous. When our diet is heavy laden in artificial chemicals and preservatives, the liver and kidneys become overloaded with detoxification and the result is often inflammation. Start reading labels when you go shopping at the grocery store. If the label contains a long list of chemicals that you probably can't pronounce, better to pass on it. The simpler the ingredient list, the better.

Where do you begin to reduce your inflammation? First, eat more fruits and vegetables. Next, reduce some of the most problematic foods listed above. Then, add some of the following beverage teas to help fight the fire, all of which are available in natural foods grocery stores:

Peppermint Leaf clears inflammation generally, but specifically in the digestive system, liver, lungs, throat, head and eyes. Peppermint oil capsules reduce the burning pain of irritable bowel syndrome (IBS).

Fresh Ginger Root can promote digestion, activate circulation and reduce pain. Lightly simmer 2 or 3 thick slices for 5-10 minutes in a pint of water. Sweeten with honey.

Turmeric Root is very anti-inflammatory, as well as improving the health of the liver and gall bladder. It is available fresh or dried. Use 1/2 teaspoon of dried powder per cup of hot water for tea.

Chrysanthemum Flowers clear fire that causes hypertension, insomnia, headaches and red painful eyes. These are used in Chinese medicine to prevent over heating in Spring and Summer.

Chamomile Flowers and **Holy Basil (Tulsi) Leaves** reduce the inflammation that leads to agitated emotions and anxiety and help us to cultivate calmness. My favorite tea is a blend from Organic India called "Sweet Rose Tulsi Tea." It makes a wonderful heat quenching ice tea, and the scent of roses takes me to a very peaceful rose garden where I delightfully chill out.

CHAPTER 4

Kirin's Finger Is Saved!

WE SAVED MY niece Kirin's index finger with herbs, love and the grace of God. My sister called me right after the accident happened to her daughter at the factory where she worked. The malfunctioning machine chewed up two fingers and her thumb. The doctor said that he sewed Kirin's index finger back on, "Because it was the merciful thing to do." He didn't think there was much chance if it living. Enter the stars: Tienchi, Aloe Vera and Arnica. Now it is 6 weeks since the accident. Yesterday the merciful doctor, with amazement, declared that this is now a viable finger. She grew a large amount of skin to cover the bare tendon in just the past week. A+ to Kirin and her herb friends for such a great job of healing! This is why I became an herbalist. The joys are many. So, who are these finger saving herbs?

Tienchi (aka San Qi) was the first Chinese herb I befriended. My ex-husband Charlie was a martial artist and herbalist who introduced me to it for both bleeding and bruising. Magical and life saving, it is the primary herb used in Traditional Asian medicines for traumatic injuries. There is one form of it that is commercially available here called Yunnan Bai Yao. During the Vietnam War, for about a decade, we were unable to obtain this herb because it was included in all of the Viet Cong soldiers' medicine packs. In addition to stopping bleeding inside and outside, Tienchi relieves pain and shock. The old packages included "gunshot wounds" as one of the conditions it treats. The Latin names of Tienchi (San Qi) are Panax notoginseng or Panax pseudoginseng. It is in the large Araliaceae plant family, which includes ginseng varieties, but this herb is very different in action. Kirin is making tea with Tienchi powder daily.

The first time I personally realized how powerful Tienchi could be, I severely cut my finger on a piece of broken glass I didn't see in the dishpan. After applying a compress for 10 minutes, the bleeding was not slowing down and I was getting woozy. About that time my herbalist husband comes in and saves the day with Tienchi. He packed the powdered herb on my cut and applied pressure with a guaze. Honest to God – within a minute or two, the bleeding stopped! We wrapped it with a bandage and left it for 24 hours. I was amazed the next day to see that the wound had begun closing so well in one day. Herbs truly save lives.

Aloe Vera was the second hero. Kirin has been drinking the juice since the beginning and as the bandages came off, she could use it topically. The exposed tendon needs to be kept "wet" with special bandages. We added Aloe Vera to that treatment, applying it every bandage change. Aloe Vera is widely available in many forms. It is renown for treating burns (I prefer Manuka honey for burns), cuts and abrasions, in part for its reliable delivery of oxygen to the cells, essential in saving a finger. Aloe Vera heals the mucosa of the gastro-intestinal tract, and is often used for chronic dry bowel movements. This succulent is easy to grow in pots.

Arnica was another remedy that my sister used right away. This flower is toxic as a tea, but in the highly diluted homeopathic form, it is a brilliant remedy for the pain of injuries, tight muscles and bruises. Homeopathic Arnica is available in a topical gel or cream, as well as a tablet for internal ingestion, in your natural foods store.

Kirin was lucky to have a caring boyfriend who massaged her acupressure points, treating the uninjured side to help the injured side. He also has been learning about Qi Gong and ways of improving the flow of Qi (energy) and blood with breathing exercises, great for healing. And of course, her beloved dog, Lola, has been by Kirin's side doing her part of the healing work.

CHAPTER 5

Sugar: My Drug of Choice

THIS IS THE time of year that we all crave change for the better. A huge number of Americans resolved recently to lose weight, exercise more, and eat healthier in the new year. More than 90% will fall short of the goal before very many weeks of 2013 pass. Why? Are we weak willed? I say, no. We are addicted to bad foods, mostly sugar, fats and refined carbohydrates.

Unfortunately, this addiction is killing us very insidiously. The current generation of kids are predicted to live shorter lives than their parents, in large measure due to the epidemic of obesity and diabetes in children these days, with 1/3 of Americans kids and 2/3 of adults now overweight or obese. This number has been rising since 1980, when high fructose corn syrup became widely used in our foods and drinks. Sugar in all of its forms is very addictive, activating the same brain centers as cocaine, causing the release of dopamine and a feeling of euphoria. Just like other drugs, frequent sugar eaters develop a tolerance and need larger quantities to feel good. Recent research shows that fructose in particular, never appears to register "enough" in the brain, so we keep eating more. That is also a problem with the artificial sweeteners which cause us to eat more calories in an attempt to "fill in" what is missing calorically with that extreme sweet taste. Do our lives lack sweetness?

Table sugar (aka sucrose) is made from sugar beets or sugar cane. It is composed of ½ fructose and ½ glucose. In the 70's a cheap sweetener was developed from the subsidized corn crops, and high fructose corn syrup was born (aka Karo Syrup). This human creation is 55% fructose and 45% glucose. Even though the different forms of sugar have the same amount of calories, they are metabolized differently.

I, personally, do not eat corn or corn products. About 15 years ago I learned that caterpillars of monarch butterflies were dying in large numbers from exposure to genetically modified (GM) corn pollen, growing beside their favorite weed, milkweed. If GM corn pollen is killing caterpillars, can corn be a healthy food for humans? Anyhow, that was when my corn ban began. Unfortunately, now the corn all around the world has been polluted by the GM corn seeds that are widely distributed. Seed producers high in the mountains of central Mexico, for generations have grown many unique varieties of maize, but even these no longer are pure strains of corn. For you animal lovers, read labels: corn should not be fed to dogs or cats (or cattle) as it leads to digestive and skin problems. Part of our global warming problem is that the feedlot cows are being quickly fattened up on corn which makes them fart a dangerous amount of methane gas for our fragile environment.

The average American eats over 130 pounds of sugar per year. That is 1/3 of a pound of sugar per day! The scientific community is recognizing that in those quantities, sugar is toxic. There is a very interesting lecture on YouTube called "Sugar: The Bitter Truth" by Dr Robert Lustig. He talks about a study they did with college kids for 2 weeks, in which they controlled their sugar intake completely. After establishing a baseline of blood values on a low sugar diet, 25% of their calories were replaced by sugary drinks, made with high fructose corn syrup. In only 2 weeks, the students experienced significant increases in their very low density cholesterol numbers (VLDL). These VDLD are truly the bad guys who cause cardiovascular disease. The liver is unable to convert the sugar fast enough and converts it instead to bad fats.

So why do we love sweets so much? In Nature no food that contains fructose is poisonous. Evolutionarily speaking, the sweet flavor tells us we are making a safe food choice. But, we used to get fructose primarily from fruit, mixed with fiber which slows absorption, and eating whole fruits limits consumption. Now with fructose separated from its other natural components and consumed in such large quantities, it has become a wolf in sheep's clothing: we remember "safe" but this is a dangerous fake. When we went through the "low-fat foods craze" a while ago, the fats were replaced with sugars. No wonder heart disease, diabetes, and obesity continued to rise.

Cancer is another concern for we sugar addicts. There is a significant decrease in risk with limiting sugar consumption. Sugar causes the body to produce insulin which fuels some types of cancers, in particular, breast and colon, in which the tumors have insulin receptors, so that cupcake goes straight to the tumor to help it grow. For cancer patients it is important to avoid all of the forms that sugar takes: wine and other alcohols, white flour products, white sugar, brown sugar, and high fructose corn syrup. These are all ultimately processed as sugar, producing an increase in insulin. Sugar creates an inflammatory response in the body and most health problems will worsen with this increase in inflammation.

Usually sweets provide emotional comfort. I do not have the answer to this challenge, but I have found some guidelines that have helped me with my sweet tooth. Read labels for starters. If sugar** is near the top of the list, leave it. If I have sweets, I make them. That way I have control over how much and which kind of sugar I use, and reserve this for special occasions only. Even the healthy choices in sweeteners can be over done, so I use sparingly honey, maple syrup, agave syrup, and coconut nectar. I also have been experimenting with the herb stevia as a sweetener. Mostly, I rely on fruit for my sweet treats. Sometimes a big craving for sweets can signal a protein deficiency, so be sure to explore that possibility. For me, when I crave sweets, usually it is my little inner child wanting comfort. Now I sit, breathe, relax and hope the craving passes soon....Once I get to about the "3 weeks without sugar point", it will get a little easier, just like changing any other bad habit. The goal is progress, not perfection.

**Sugars usually end in -ose: sucrose, glucose, fructose, maltose, dextrose, lactose, etc.

References:

Food, Inc. - a documentary about the current state of food production in US, including factory farming and GMO's.

Food Rules: An Eater's Manual by Michael Pollan – a sensible guide to making mindful, responsible food choices.

CHAPTER 6

Winter Solstice: Longer Days Are On the Way

HERE IN THE mountains of southern California, winter has arrived. Frosty nights, cold winds and rainy weather are all part of our version of winter. Between now and December 22, the Winter Solstice, the days will continue to get shorter. I never get used to having darkness come before 5 PM, but soon, each day will give us about 90 seconds longer daylight. For those who are super sensitive to the darkness, winter time depression can be a problem. There are some very effective lights that you can purchase to supplement the missing sunlight until the real thing again arrives in abundance.

Winter is the season associated with the Kidney/Bladder organ system, according to Traditional Chinese Medicine. The "Chinese Kidney" encompasses the endocrine system, the adrenals, the reproductive organs, bones, ears and the brain, as well as the water circulating organs, the kidneys and bladder. Strengthening the Kidney can benefit all of the associated components, whether it is done with foods, herbs, visualizations, or directed exercises such as Qi Gong, Tai Qi, or Yoga.

Dark colored foods strengthen the Kidney system. This includes foods like blueberries, blackberries, raspberries, cranberries, cherries, seaweeds, dark leafy greens, black and wild rice, black beans, and black sesame seeds. The salty flavor found in miso, soy sauce and fish, will also guide foods into the Kidneys. Be careful if you have hypertension or edema, however, when it comes to increasing the salty flavor in your foods. Animal proteins are also generally suggested for strengthening the Kidneys. Lamb, beef, chicken, turkey, trout, salmon and shrimp will provide the most warming properties. Pork is cooling and moistening for the Kidney.

Winter is the time for building up our reserves and conserving our energy. Root vegetable soups and stews help us do this. Roots are the plants' food storage units which can also benefit us. Use a little more warming spices in winter dishes to counteract the cold environment outside. This may include things like curry, onions, garlic, hot peppers, cumin, fennel seeds, rosemary, parsley, ginger, cinnamon and cloves.

Here is a very easy **Creamy Curry Soup** to prepare on a cold winter night:

Steam a vegetable (or mixture of vegetables) like broccoli, cauliflower, carrots, sweet potato or onions until soft.

Put the soft veggies, the steam water, and a can of low fat coconut milk in the blender, then return to the stove and heat thoroughly.

Season to taste with curry powder and sea salt (or miso or soy sauce). Garnish with fresh parsley.

Enjoy with whole grain bread or crackers and voila, a fast, delicious, healthy winter meal in about 10 minutes!

CHAPTER 7

Year of the Dragon: Chinese New Year

JANUARY 23, 2012 began the Chinese New Year under the influence of Dragon energy. Knowing what that is can help us to act accordingly to maintain health and sanity. In Chinese astrology, there are 12 animal signs that rotate through time yearly in the following order: rat, ox, tiger, rabbit, dragon, snake, horse, sheep, monkey, rooster, dog, and pig. The New Year begins on the new moon at the end of January or beginning of February, and the traditional celebration, the Spring Festival, continues two weeks until the full moon, emphasizing home, family and food. We are soon leaving the Year of the Rabbit. Depending on your birth sign, how your animal sign and the calendar animal get along influences what that year may bring for you. I am a Tiger, and since Dragons and Tigers are both control freaks, I best lay low and not be my usual bossy self for the next 12 months or I may come up against some serious opposition. When 2013 rolls around and it becomes the Year of the Snake, it will be easier to resume my old ways.

Dragons are magnificent creatures, as are the years they influence. They are confident, dynamic, charismatic, feisty, vibrant, noble-hearted, healthy and gifted with power and luck. In their worst moments they are ruthless, demanding, opinionated, egocentric, willful and pompous. Under that fire-breathing bravado is the Dragon's soft under belly which is tender hearted and endowed with the highest of moral character. With that type of energy, 2012 will surely be a memorable year. Each of the 5 Elements (Water, Wood, Fire, Earth and Metal) also influences the year. 2012 will be the year of the Water Dragon. That Water energy will bring out friendships, love and creativity.

Health wise, the important considerations we should all have in the Dragon year ahead of us are to:

1) Curb indulgences and excesses. Dragons like to party.

2) Find activities that cultivate calmness, such as meditation, yoga, breathing exercises, Tai Qi, or gentle walks in nature. This will protect us from the flames of the Dragon.

3) Maintain a gentle diet so that the body does not become agitated and over heated.

4) Remember the importance of rest to balance activity. Overdoing can lead to stress, a common problem for Dragons.

There are some interesting customs that I have adopted over the decades around Chinese New Year. I clean house the day before to sweep out all of the unwanted remnants of the last year, but not on New Year's Day...you don't want to sweep away the accumulating good energy of the new cycle. Chinese New Year's Eve celebrations always include lots of yummy foods, leading to pretty severe food stagnation indigestion by the time the New Year arrives. The Chinese medicine pills called Bao He Wan OR hawthorn berry tea are traditional "nightcaps" after the day of over eating too many different foods. These have also become mainstays in my home post Thanksgiving and other feasts.

My hope for this magnificent Dragon year is that we may all connect with our highest selves and harness this powerful Dragon energy to make significant changes in ourselves and the troubled world around us. I recently watched a remarkable documentary about doing just that, called *I Am*, by Tom Shadyac, writer, producer and director, of some of our favorite comedy movies. He learned about generosity from his beloved father, who, along with Danny Thomas, started the St. Jude's Children's Hospital, which treats all seriously sick kids, whether they can pay for it or not. *I Am* will help you become a believer that your little contributions towards good do indeed make this planet a better place for all of us to live. Happy New Year!

CHAPTER 8

Pet Remedies

MY FAMILY INCLUDES four cats and four dogs. I, personally, cannot imagine life without animals. Their unconditional love and devotion provide comfort for so many of us. Taking care of their physical needs begins with a breed specific, appropriate diet. Dogs are omnivores, meaning they eat basically everything. Cats are carnivores, meat eaters. In my uninformed days of youth, I made the mistake of feeding my animals a vegetarian diet, similar to mine. Dogs, and especially cats, are not designed to be vegetarians. Cats are extremely sensitive to herbs, drugs and foods, so much care must be taken to protect them. Never give an alcohol tincture to a cat or dog, whose livers lacks the ability to detoxify alcohol. Both cats and dogs, similarly, cannot process chocolate or caffeine, as well as the artificial sweetener, Xylitol.

Human medications can be deadly for cats and dogs, as well. Cleaning products and house plants can also pose lethal threats to our furry family. For more information call the ASPCA Animal Poison Control Center at (888)426-4435.

Some of the prohibited foods for dogs include:

1. Grapes and Raisins – even small amounts can cause vomiting and kidney failure
2. Avocados – fruit, peel and leaves all contain persin, toxic in large amounts.
3. Onions and Garlic – occasional small amounts are OK, but large amounts can injure red blood cells and lead to anemia.

4. Macadamia Nuts – as few a 5 or 6 macadamia nuts can be fatal, causing paralysis of the hindquarters, tremors and high fever.

5. Dairy products can cause diarrhea and digestive upset.

6. Tea, Coffee, Chocolate and other Caffeine containing foods are fatal in large amounts, with no antidote to treat the tremors, seizures, bleeding and rapid heartbeat that they cause. Little dogs are most at risk with small doses being big for them. Dark chocolate is the most dangerous, but white chocolate is not safe either.

7. Xylitol in candy, gum, toothpaste, baked goods – for dogs and cats it increases insulin, causing a severe drop in blood sugar, followed by vomiting, loss of coordination and seizures, and within a few days, liver failure.

8. Bones can splinter and injure their throats and GI tract, especially cooked bones, and never give chicken bones. Pigs' ears swell greatly in their stomachs and can cause injury.

9. Pork fat and fat trimmings can cause pancreatitis.

10. Raw Eggs and Meats may cause food poisoning (salmonella or E coli). An enzyme in raw egg whites interferes with the absorption of B vitamins.

11. Yeast dough, before rising – can cause abdominal pain and alcohol poisoning.

12. Alcoholic beverages in all forms hurt their livers.

Cats will also need to be protected from eating tuna too frequently, due to high mercury content. And, limit the amount of liver your cat gets. The vitamin A can be toxic and cause bone deformities and death. Cats should not be given raw fish, which contains an enzyme that can destroy thiamin and lead to neurological injury. As with dogs, no grapes, raisins, onions, garlic, dairy products, raw meat or raw eggs. And remember that dog food it not for cats; cat food is not for dogs.

Many of the commercial dog and cat foods, even ones sold by the vets, contain corn, soy, meat by-products, and artificial colorings and flavorings. Those are all unhealthy choices for our pets. Corn is not well tolerated by many cats and dogs, and can contribute to allergies and ill health. Soy commonly causes digestive upset in both cats and dogs. The majority of corn and soy crops are genetically modified, another risk factor. Meat by-products can legally include diseased animals when it comes to making pet foods.

My cats get a mostly wet food diet, with a little kibble on the top to clean their teeth, and primarily meat, with very little grain. My dogs get a mixture of salmon and sweet potato kibble and homemade chicken soup. Each week I cook together chicken thighs, rice and a variety of vegetables, including squash, string beans, sweet potatoes, cabbage, carrots, parsley and other greens. They have thrived since puppyhood on this mixture. Homemade peanut butter biscuits and dried slices of duck or chicken, round out their doggy cuisine. BE CAREFUL: don't buy dried poultry from China. It has been found to be contaminated with antibiotics that are toxic to dogs.

I don't often treat my cats with herbs or supplements, due to the difficulty with which it is to get herbs into them. Between their finicky palates and their unwillingness to let me shove a pill into their throats, I usually have to rely on vet visits for the cats, with a few exceptions. The dogs, on the other hand, are easy to doctor with herbs, either put into a tasty food, or put into the back of their throats in capsule form. Some of my favorite remedies include:

FISH OR FLAX OIL – this is an essential supplement for any dog with allergic skin issues.

HUANG LIAN SU PILLS – these contain an extract of one herb, Coptis/ Huang Lian. Internally they treat diarrhea and gastritis. Topically, they can be dissolved in hot water and used to wash wounds. The dissolved tablets can be strained through a coffee filter and used as an eyewash, very effective for those kitten eye infections that are so common.

SLIPPERY ELM POWDER – this herb soothes an irritated gut and normalizes the bowels.

BACH'S RESCUE REMEDY FOR PETS – homeopathic remedy for shock.

CALMS FORTE TABLETS – this homeopathic remedy calms frightened animals.

LAVENDER OIL – rub a few drops on your hands and then apply around the chest to a dog who is nervous or anxious.

TIENCHI (SAN QI) POWDER – apply to cuts to stop bleeding.

CALENDULA OR DANDELION TEA – good to wash wounds.

References:

The Complete Holistic Dog Book by Drs Allegretti and Sommers

4 Paws, 5 Directions by Dr Schwartz

The New Natural Cat by Anitra Frazier

Dr Pitcairn's Guide to Natural Pet Care by Dr Pitcairn

Chinese Herbal Formulas for Veterinarians by Drs Chen, Chen, Beebe, and Salewski

CHAPTER 9

Tyler's 40 Day Vision Quest

THERE IS A reading in the Taoist book of wisdom, *The I Ching*, called "The Arousing Force of Thunder" which states that the purpose of thunder in our lives is to arouse and awaken us. Thunder comes in the springtime when all life is renewed to awaken the hibernating creatures. The shock provides a time of growth, development and awe, and is sometimes necessary to disrupt complacency. Calmness is always necessary in dealing with the shock. If one's energy is scattered or disordered, one will be easily jolted by every shock that comes along. But one who is centered will act appropriately, regardless of what confronts her. Those who are stimulated and awakened by thunder channel its power to aid in their quest for truth, resulting in spiritual development within. One who receives this hexagram should reflect upon her chosen path, stage of spiritual growth and spiritual patterns which she accepts. Such patterns determine who one really is. This hexagram was the answer that I was given when I asked, "Why did I lose my Tyler during the July 4th fireworks?"

This was the most painful, shocking and difficult time of my life to date. I have never prayed, meditated and cried so much. I wanted Tyler back more than I have ever wanted anything. It was torture to feel his pain. For the first three weeks I barely ate or slept, and spent every non-working moment walking, riding my bike or driving the area in the search for my lost companion. Some of my friends expressed concern over my obsession to find Tyler, and those who were discouraging my pursuit had to be avoided. Thank God for the wonderful support and encouragement that I received from animal communicators, psychics and intuitive friends who all said that Tyler was alive, disoriented and scared.

My veterinarian friends, John and Priscella Limehouse suggested that I contact Janet Goldman to communicate with Tyler. She and her husband were enormously helpful. I was asked to provide a map of my area, his picture and biography. They not only provided me with guidance on where to search for him, but reassured me that he was alive. In my panic they provided me with calm guidance. Janet revealed to me his history of abuse and the shock of the fireworks had him stuck in those painful and fearful memories. He lacked the trust to allow anyone to help him. I was told to send him the memory of my scent and the vision of coming home to me. Since he left I had been sending him a tunnel of protective golden light from my heart through which he could safely pass. My concern was that Tyler was not streetwise and would have to cross a busy highway to come home. Janet told me on day five that he was confined in a dark cement-like structure which was cool and damp, and could not muster up the courage to back out. This was near a basketball court and playground. I finally figured out it must have been the drain tunnel across the highway from my house running in front of a school. I camped out there with food and his tennis ball and thought I heard a weak whimper coming from inside. Day 7 a friend named Max came to fix my washing machine and eagerly offered to crawl through the quarter-mile tunnel. What outstanding friends I am blessed to have. Neither the Fire Department nor animal regulation groups were willing to accept the liability for an animal stuck in the tunnel. A child would have been a different story. For me, Tyler's life was as precious as a child's.

The search proved fruitless. However, Max convinced me to go look at a Border Collie who desperately needed help out of a bad living situation with an attacking Chow. He had her brother and sister, and knew she and I would be a beautiful match. The moment that Sheba Dove and I met it was love at first sight, exactly like Tyler and I connected seven years ago at the pound. Of course I would give her the home she deserved. Now I had a companion to help me in my nightlong searching for Tyler. Sheba Dove is one of the most affectionate animals that I have ever known, so I think it would be correct to say that she rescued me with her kisses and cuddles. She adores me, and I'm guessing that I am the first one who has ever truly loved her. Unlike all of her siblings and parents who are predominantly black, Sheba is white like a dove with the silkiest coat I've ever touched. She soothed my pain in so many ways.

One of the lessons that has been profound for me through this has been forgiveness. I was enraged at the previous owners of Tyler who had instilled such profound fear. I had to learn to forgive them for their ignorance. I was also extremely angry at my friend Michael, who was supposed to be watching him that night. Michael turned out to be an incredible support who looked for Tyler almost as many hours as did I. His profound love for me and for Tyler helped teach me the power of forgiveness. We cried on one another's shoulders and provided tenderness through the harsh experience of loss and disappointment. What a powerful blessing.

Into the second week of searching for Tyler another animal communicator, Connie Adams, suggested that I write a list of what I was willing to do to get him back and for everything I was doing, list what I expected the universe or God to provide. So for instance, I put up 150 color flyers of Tyler and asked that the universe let someone see one who had seen him. I think all of Ojai knows Tyler by now. The next day she asked me what came up for me in this exercise. Clearly the answer was that I lacked trust that the universe would provide. Trust. Tyler and I were going through a similar set of fears due to our lack of trust. It was at this point that I think a spiritual awakening began to unfold for me. For many years I had lost sight of the God within me which is always guiding and instructing me. I was taking all the credit for my achievements. Spiritually I had become very cynical and uninspired. My dear friend, Lynn, reminded me that Tyler had given me gifts by his loss, one of which was a reawakening of my spirituality. Another was that in my intense strength of purpose to find him, those who were not supportive of my mission, squelching my hopes, had to be avoided. I had to refuse negative influences and stay strong. Janet had advised me to move slowly and be calm and peaceful to help Tyler find his way home and that I constantly practiced.

Week 3 Tyler was seen in the night by my friend Pam who helped me so much in the physical search. That day one of her massage clients had died in her arms, and she could not sleep that night. So as she walked the neighborhood processing her grief, off in the distance was Tyler. Still too freaked out to trust anyone he ran. Week 4 was getting really tough on me. Janet saw him still alive and on the move. This renewed my hope. This past week I must have had a radar signal up for lost dogs and helped 3 return home who showed up at my house. One was a old disoriented German Shorthair whose mate had just died. Buddy was running full boar towards the highway when I called to him and he stopped. His owner said he hadn't been eating and kept wandered around lost. Heidi, the Doberman, was escaping her uncaring dog-sitter, and the Pomeranian just could not find her way home.

One of my students suggested that I contact a psychic named Pam Oslie for more help. Normally it takes 9-12 months to get an appointment with her. Pam called me the next day and again assured me that Tyler was alive and too skittish to accept help. She saw a tall woman and older man that could potentially help him. She feared that he was moving North towards coyote country, away from people, and would be too tired and weak to run from them. She saw his blue collar with my phone number still on him, but said he had traveled out of the local area. She told me to sternly tell him to go to a road or home and let someone help him. She said let him know that they will call me and I will pick you up in the car. Part 2 of her instruction was to ask the angels to guide him to this safe older woman who would help him, not hurt him. For the next 10 days this became my constant thought, meditation and prayer. Pam also told me that I had no idea how many angels, guides and beings were assisting me in reuniting with Tyler.

Then, the happiest day of my life came, 40 days after Tyler ran away. Bernice, the tall, gray-haired woman called with my Tyler at her house. She lives on the edge of the Los Padres National Forest, 6 or 7 miles from my house. He had scratched on her back door late that night asking for help. The angels guided him to her, and because of the gentleness of her and her husband, he trusted them. My prayers were answered and my trust in God reaffirmed. As you might guess our reunion was one of ecstatic joy. Tyler was covered with tics (about 100 to be exact), his tired swollen feet were bloody with foxtails, but he was alive and in great shape. He had lost 17 pounds and fortunately left on the chubby side so could afford the loss of weight. He came back not only thinner, but wiser and stronger, having faced his profound fears for 40 days and 40 nights. I too lost about 17 pounds and gained strength and wisdom that I never dreamed possible.

Thank you Tyler for the gifts you gave me in this tremendous spiritual awakening. I am eternally grateful to all the helpers that facilitated this process.

Cathy McNease - August 1997

I adopted Tyler from the Ojai Humane Society as an abused puppy in 1990. After his magical return to me in 1997, he lived another six years as my devoted companion. The last couple years of his life he developed diabetes, needing twice daily insulin shots and went blind from the disease. Yet, he never stopped being that loving and caring dog that came into my life many years before. Tyler died in my arms at 13 when his kidneys finally failed. He has continued to be my guardian angel dog.

I can't help but wonder if my new puppy, Pepper, was guided into my life by my angel, Tyler. They have such similar dispositions. Again, the Ojai Humane Society has provided me with this lovely canine companion. For this I am very grateful. If I calculated correctly, Pepper was born on Thanksgiving Day, 2007. Serendipity!

C McN

March 2008

I have adopted a lovely puppy companion for Pepper. Her name is Ginger. I don't recognize her, but I am sure Pepper does. They adore each other! Pepper helped me pick out which puppy to bring home from the shelter. Ginger's birthday is very close to mine. I am truly blessed, as are Pepper and Ginger. As time has passed, I am positive that Pepper is the return of my beloved Tyler; they have such similar mannerisms and the same eyes.

C McN

May 2008

My pack has expanded with the addition of Tansy, a one year old Maltese/ Poodle who was purchased at 12 weeks by my patient for her children. When one of them developed allergies to her, Tansy was given to an abusive MD and her daughter. Fortunately, an angel of mercy delivered her into my care after only a couple of months of poor treatment. She and Ginger have become best friends! All the dogs play nicely together and give me great joy to watch.

C McN

April 2010

My pack is now completed by the happy go lucky boy named Clover. He too is a Poodle/Maltese that I saw in the Ojai paper being offered by a Maltese rescuer in Santa Paula. Tansy had nothing to do with him for 9 days, growling if he got too close. He didn't give up...now they are buddies! He joined our family July 3, 2011, at almost 4 months old. Clover is now 1 1/2 and continues to want to play non-stop!

CMcN

Sept 2012

CHAPTER 10

Remembering My Parents

Margaret Evelyn (Witmer) McNease
Born 11-2-20 in Goshen, Indiana
Died 12-25-99 in South Bend, Indiana

MOM DIED ON Christmas day, just as Dad, my brother, Mark, and I sat down for Christmas dinner. Caro, our sister, had stayed at the bedside because her breathing seem a bit rough. Before we took a bite, Caro came in to announce that Mom was gone. I remember watching Dad unravel, whaling, "What am I gonna do without her?" Even 50 years together wasn't enough. We didn't expect Dad to live a year, but he soldiered on for 10 years, always a little down, at best. They had remained lovebirds for 50 years.

Dad vowed never to celebrate Christmas again, and promptly sent me sixteen huge cartons of Christmas decorations, including the whole Santa and his reindeer roof display. Goodwill got most of it, but I kept the lights and some treasures, neatly contained in 2 boxes. Every year I take them out and look at all the stuff that reminds me of Mom and how much her piano students loved her. Many of the Christmas treasures that I saved were gifts from them. My mother was one of the most generous people that I have ever known. She showed me the example of always giving what you can to those who are in need. I loved that about her.

Mom loved animals and often rescued strays that she nursed back to health. My grandma, Non, told me that when Mom was a little girl, she told people that when she grew up she was going to start an orphanage for cats and dogs. I saw her risk her life on numerous occasions helping a lost or hurt animal out of traffic. The apple didn't fall far from the tree with my animal family of eight. I do so love living with animals nearby.

Mom lived life with gusto. She had fire red passion. If you ever heard her play the piano, you experienced that passion. She and Dad remained in love for half of a century. They were always affectionate. As kids, it was not uncommon to hear their passion from behind closed doors. My later comfort in enjoying sex and experiencing passion, were my take away gifts from their loving example, not that I have ever really had a healthy relationship. But we were not an affectionate family, just Mom and Dad. As Mark always said, their music business was their first born, and that got much of their attention. Fortunately, we all had a nanny of sorts to provide nurturing. For me it was Christine, my best friend as a child. Verna May, Christine's sister, helped with Caro, and Mark relied on Mrs. Myers, our remarkable cleaning lady.

For years I had a chip on my shoulder that Mom didn't like/want/care for me, so she left me unattended much of the time. In maturity, I came to understand that she was the perfect mother for me because she helped to cultivate my fiercely independent and courageous spirit. I am eternally grateful for that. At 63, I regularly talk to Christine on the phone, and treasure the stories about my mom. Christine was Mom's dear friend and piano student from ages 6 until 14, when she became my surrogate mom. My mother was a Scorpio with all of the predictable passion, intensity, mystery and secrets. How grateful I am that she was my mom.

Merry Christmas, Mom. I miss talking to you late at night.

Emmett Hildren (Mac) McNease
Born 11-28-23 in Prentiss, Mississippi
Died 11-13-09 in South Bend, Indiana

My dad was a lion among men. He could fix anything. My heart aches missing him. I could always call Dad with my successes and my failures and be supported, encouraged and loved. He was my "go to guy" when I needed help with money, men and life. Although I broke his heart moving to California, a year later when I left my husband, Jim, and lived out of my business, my father called me every day for several months, always ending the call with, "Keep your chin up, Baby." Dad was always so proud of my accomplishments and bragged to his friends about his California daughter, the "herb doctor."

A couple of years before he died, Alzheimer's had begun to steal his mind and his memories. We still talked, but it began to shift into me being the adult and him being the child. I miss my strong, powerful, kind friend who was also my dad. I remember him calling me, pissed off at Caro for taking his car keys away, with his secret plan. He had secured $20,000. and just needed a ride to the car dealership to pick up his purchase. Yikes! I called my sister to intercept the plan, but this was how it was with Dad and me. We felt safe sharing our secrets with each other. Even in his dementia, he knew I was safe. Of course, I had my share of secrets that I never revealed to him (it must be my Scorpio moon), like around my debts. I never wanted to look as bad off financially as I was, since making money was such an important measure of worth for him, the self made man who rose up from poverty.

But matters of the heart, problems with men, I could bare my soul with Dad. And he never gave me a hard time for saying "fuck" or anything else. The only thing we really couldn't say in our house was "ain't" because it was "too hillbilly." Dad's shame about growing up in a poor farmer's family in Mississippi never left him. If fact, by the time the dementia had really taken hold, he had re-written his past and believed that his dad was a successful banker in Ohio. He lived through World War II and the Battle of the Bulge, but couldn't face his poor, Southern past.

I miss my dad so much. He always had my back. At almost 63, I have come to resemble him in many ways, besides my strong willed stubbornness. Hip pain. Content to sit. Love of dogs. Love of flowers. Love of beauty. Love of peace and quiet. I wish my brother and sister could have known the sensitive side of dad, that I think they missed. His strength was not easy for Mark and Caro. For me, it was my wing of safety, and example that I could do or be anything I set my mind to. I don't think they saw Dad's vulnerability, which he showed to me from time to time, maybe because I was the oldest, or maybe it was because we were kindred spirits. We really understood each other. Christine told me recently that

Mom took her frustrations toward Dad out on me because I was so much like him. That explains a lot.

Happy Birthday, Dad. I miss picking out a beautiful floral calendar for you, like I did for several decades. Mark and I both remembered your birthday with email exchanges.

Appendix 1

For Practitioners of Traditional Chinese Medicine

These notes will help you in choosing foods for your patient, based on your Zang-Fu diagnosis of imbalances. I have presented this information at several acupuncture colleges in Southern California in recent years. A version of this class is available for viewing at the Lotus Institute of Integrative Medicine (eLotus.org).

HARMONIZING WITH THE SUN AND THE MOON: USING FOODS AND HERBS ACCORDING TO TRADITIONAL CHINESE NUTRITION FOR BALANCE

Course description:
This course will apply the principles of Traditional Chinese Nutrition to choosing foods to harmonize with the seasons of the year, phases of the menstrual cycle and individual constitutions. Foods and herbs for general balancing will be discussed, as well as groups of foods for specific Zang-Fu disharmonies, common patient complaints and female disorders. Cooking Chinese "food" herbs into delicious dishes will also be covered with sample dishes provided.

Sun Si Miao is considered "the father of TCM dietary therapy". He lived during the Tang Dynasty, from 590-692 AD, starting life as a very sickly child. His family sought common foods to restore their son's health since they were too poor to afford expensive herbs. In his famous book *Prescriptions Worth 1000 Pieces of Gold*, he categorized the properties and applications of many fruits, vegetables, grains, fowl, animals, fish and insects. He discussed desirable and undesirable foods for specific illnesses. His concept of dietary therapy was further developed in later works by doctors who followed in Sun Si Miao's footsteps.

A truly good doctor finds out the cause of a disease, and based on such finding, he first tries to treat it with foods. Only when foods fail to produce the desired result does he resort to medication. – Sun Si Miao

Overview of Chinese Nutrition

<u>Energetics of foods</u>: similar to looking at energetics of herbs
—temperature —flavor–direction–organ/channel affinity

<u>Use of the Five Flavors of Foods:</u>

Salty – yin – downward and inward: moistens, softens, detoxifies, regulate fluids by strengthening Kidney; counteracts hardening of muscles and glands
    Sour – yin – inward: stimulates contraction, absorption, astringency; stimulates secretions from gall bladder and pancreas; counteracts fatty foods
Bitter – yin – downward: dries and drains; reduces excess; disperses obstructions; usually clears heat; small amounts may stimulate appetite
Sweet – yang – upward: tonifies, harmonizes, moistens; builds Yin; relaxes
Full sweet (complex carbohydrates): energizing yet relaxing.
Empty sweet (fruit juice, sugar): less warming and tonifying + may agitate instead of relax the nervous system. Strongly generate dampness.
Pungent (Acrid) – yang – upward and outward: disperses stagnations of Qi, Blood and fluids; stimulates digestion; disperses external pathogens and phlegm

<u>Age/Constitutional Types:</u>

Need to match the energy of the diet with the energetic needs of the patient
Age: Infants and young children – weak middle burner
Adolescents- can tend towards heat and damp
Adults – variety in moderation (constitution should guide choices)
Elderly – weakening middle burner and waning Kidney
Constitutional type:–Excess / –Deficient
–Hot / –Cold
–Dry / –Damp

Western/Eastern Nutrition Comparisons:

–Proteins (meat, fish, eggs, beans, dairy products)
TONIFYING QI-BLOOD-YANG-YIN
–Complex carbohydrates (grains, root vegetables, beans)
TONIFYING QI (some BLOOD)
HIGH FIBER=MOVING QI (some BLOOD)
–Fats (nuts, seeds, avocados, oils, animal fats)
TONIFY YIN (some BLOOD, some QI)
MOISTEN BODY AND BOWELS
–Water (fruits, watery veggies like squash, tomatoes)
GENERATE BODY FLUIDS
–Vitamins, Minerals
VARIABLE – TONIFY, CALM
–Other chemical compounds i.e. chlorophyll; anti-oxidants like lycopene; bioflavonoids
VARIABLE – TONIFY, CLEAR HEAT/TOXINS

TCM Energetics of Food Groups:

VEGETABLES are an essential part of a healthy diet. In general the vegetables provide components to cleanse the body of toxins, regulate the Qi and benefit the blood. Those with a predominantly sweet flavor, such as sweet potatoes and carrots will tonify the Qi. Those with a slightly bitter flavor will be more effective in clearing heat and toxins and drying dampness. The fibrous vegetables such as those in the cabbage family (cabbage, broccoli, cauliflower, kale), and the spicy ones from the onion family (onions, garlic, leeks, chives) will regulate the Qi. The dark leafy green vegetables are rich in minerals which will tonify the blood. In general the vegetables are more easily digested if they are lightly cooked. Many of the vegetables have a cooling energy which can be moderated by cooking them or adding warming spices such as ginger, garlic, chives, fennel, basil or other western cooking herbs, most of which are warming. Sea vegetables will be particularly nutritious, containing abundant supplies of minerals. All seaweeds are cooling with the least cooling varieties being nori and dulse.

FRUITS contain a large proportion of water. Thus, they are particularly good for generating fluids and promoting bowel movements. Fruits digest easily and quickly and in general are best eaten alone. The sweet fruits and dried fruits such as grapes, bananas, dates and raisins have a tendency to generate dampness. The strong sour flavored fruits such as lemon, lime and grapefruit, can be used to regulate the Liver Qi. Fruits in general will have a cooling energy which can be moderated by baking with spices like cinnamon and ginger. Fruit juices are very concentrated so they should be diluted with water and consumed in moderation. Fruits are particularly beneficial in the summer months to rehydrate us and prevent summer heat conditions.

GRAINS were the first cultivated foods, providing essential nutrients for human development. Grains are Qi tonics, notably present in the sweet flavor. Most grains will be close to neutral in their energies, and are often used as a base to dispense medicinal herbs, i.e. an herb porridge (congee, jook or gruel). The grains can be pan roasted prior to cooking them to provide a more warming energy. As the grains tonify the Spleen Qi they will in most cases also eliminate dampness. Wheat is the exception because of the fact that it nourishes Yin. With grains remember to be careful with gluten-sensitive patients (wheat, rye, barley, spelt, kamut) and those who do not process carbohydrates efficiently. According to Dr Christiane Northrup, many women over 50 would be in this latter group, contributing to easy weight gain in peri- and post-menopause.

BEANS, or legumes, are Qi tonics which in general are good to promote urination and bowel movements. Their drying nature can be offset by the addition of sea vegetables, oil or salt. Soy beans and black beans both nourish Yin, and are the exceptions to the overall drying nature of beans. The concentrated nutrients in beans can be difficult to digest. The smaller beans, such as peas, adukis and lentils are more easily digested. Beans are rendered more easily digested if the soaking water is discarded; they are well cooked; and fennel, cumin, epasote, seaweed or vinegar are added to the cooking process.

NUTS AND SEEDS contain large amounts of oils and essential fatty acids which can be useful in lubricating the bowels, nourishing the skin and benefitting the nervous system. They are also tonifying to the Qi and Blood, noted in the sweet flavor. Because of their high oil content nuts and seeds can easily become rancid if not properly stored. Once hulled, they should be refrigerated to maximize their shelf life. Nuts can be difficult to digest. This can be moderated by roasting or soaking prior to use. Because they are very concentrated foods, nuts and seeds should be eaten in moderation and chewed well.

ANIMAL PRODUCTS will be the strongest foods to tonify Qi and Blood. They are clearly indicated in deficiency conditions, and should be limited in excess conditions. Lamb, beef and chicken will be the most warming for the Yang. Fish will usually be milder in tonifying properties with the oily fish, like salmon and sardines, moistening Yin and Blood. Shellfish, most notably crab and shrimp, should be limited by those with serious Liver imbalances because they are believed to generate internal wind. All fish should be chosen carefully, choosing ones that are abundant, well managed and caught or farmed in environmentally friendly ways, as well as avoiding those fish that are high in mercury and other contaminants. For complete fish lists visit: www.seafoodwatch.org. Small portions of any animal food are consumed at a time, and will be more easily digested in soups. Attention should be paid to the way in which the animals have been raised and slaughtered, avoiding those raised with antibiotics, hormones and inhumane methods. Dairy products and eggs will be particularly nourishing for Yin and Blood, however they may create dampness or phlegm if overeaten. Many individuals are allergic or sensitive to dairy products. Goat's milk and cultured cow's milk (yogurt and kefir) tend to create less sensitivity problems.

BEVERAGES: All alcoholic beverages generate heat and to some degree, dampness. Rice wine and red wine are used medicinally when we desire a warming and blood-moving substance. Caffeine containing drinks will also generate heat, with the exception of green tea which is cooling. Sodas and juices laden with sugar and chemicals generate dampness. Artificial sweeteners may burden the Liver and lead to stagnation. They may also set up a craving for sugary drinks and foods.

Brief Summary of Individual Foods:

ANIMAL PRODUCTS:

Eggs – tonify Qi, blood and Yin; secure fetus

Dairy products (from cows) – tonify Qi, blood and Yin; can create dampness

Goat's milk products – tonify Qi and blood; are warming and less allergenic than cow's milk products

Pork – moistens Yin (KD)

Beef – builds blood, tendons and bones, reduce dampness (SP)

Chicken – builds blood, replenish Jing (LV)

Lamb – warmest meat for Yang, promote lactation (HT)

Fish (in general) – tonify Qi, drain damp (LU)

Oily fish (like salmon) – moisten Yin and blood (LU)

Shellfish (in general) – caution with internal wind conditions

Mussels – build Jing

Shrimp – warm Yang

Oysters – build Jing

GRAINS:

Wheat – nourish Yin, calm Heart, astringe fluid loss

Millet – harmonize middle burner

Rye – regulate Liver, dry damp

Oats – calm nervous system, soothe irritation on skin

Brown rice – hypoallergenic, calms Shen, tonify Qi

White rice – alleviate diarrhea

Basmati rice – aromatic, so more drying and Qi regulating

Quinoa – most Yang tonifying of "grains"
Corn – tonify and regulate Qi
Barley – soothes inflammation, reduce dampness

BEANS:

Lentil – tonify middle
Soy - moisten Yin, clear heat, promote lactation
Black - tonify Yin and Yang, benefit Kidney
Mung – clear heat and toxins, summer heat and damp-heat
Kidney – tonify Kidney
Pea – strengthen middle, promote bowel movement
Aduki (Azuki) – drain dampness, strengthen Kidney, move blood

NUTS and SEEDS:

Almond – benefit Lung, stop cough (like "Xing Ren")
Walnut – benefit Lung and Kidney, warm Yang
Pinenut – moisten Lung and Large intestine
Sunflower – relax Liver, descend Yang (greens clear Liver heat)
Sesame – nourish Yin and blood (Black ones benefit Jing)
Pumpkin – promote urination to relieve damp-heat in lower burner (for bladder or prostate); anti-parasitic

MEDICINAL MUSHROOMS benefit Qi, regulate fluids:

Shitake (xiang gu)– tonify Qi/blood, benefit immunity
Hei Mu Er (black wood ears) – move blood, reduce stagnation; contra pregnancy
Bai Mu Er (white wood ears) – nourish Yin, promote BM

VEGETABLES:

Cabbage family (in general) – regulate Qi, many clear heat

Bitter greens (in general) – clear heat, dry damp
Onion family (in general) – regulate Qi, warm Yang
Potato – nourish Yin, reduce inflammations and ulcers
Tomato – clear heat, especially from Liver; clear summer heat
Kale – heal Stomach
Cabbage – heal Stomach, long growing season=better for deficiency
Carrot – tonify Qi, benefit Liver and Lung
Beet – regulate chest Qi (like "Gua Lou"), nourish blood
Lettuce – clear heat; fast growing=better for excess
Cucumber – clear heat and inflammation; careful with dampness
Celery – soothe Liver, promote urination, regulate Qi
Parsley – promote digestion, promote urination
Spinach – nourish blood, promote BM
Garlic – warm Yang, anti-microbial; careful with heat, especially dry eyes &
mouth sores
Summer Squash – clear summer heat
Winter Squash – tonify Qi/blood
Asparagus – promote urination, clear damp-heat
Sweet Potato – tonify Qi/blood
Seaweeds – cooling, softening (kombu-most), calming, high in minerals
(wakame, hiziki-most); dulse and nori the best with cold

FRUITS:

Apple – regulate Qi, relieve depression
Banana – cold and damp, clear heat; tonify Qi
Cherry – tonify blood and Qi; good for deficiency; reduce Bi pain
Pear – transform phlegm, moisten Lung; similar to "Chuan Bei Mu"
Watermelon – clear summer heat, promote urination
Plum – regulate Liver
Citrus fruit peels – regulate Qi, dry damp
Orange – moisten dryness
Lemon – regulate Liver, clear Liver heat, detoxify

Grapefruit – regulate Liver; avoid with western pharmaceuticals

Papaya, pineapple, mango – promote digestion, but very sweet, so careful with dampness

Berries – tonify blood, moisten dryness; low-sugar fruit

Sweet vs. Sour fruits – sweet is Yang, sour is Yin, so a sour variety tends to be more cooling

Fruit juices – concentrated in sugar, so can be dampening

Dried fruits – Yin is reduced, so tend to be warmer than fresh; excess can be dampening due to concentration of sugar

Cooking with Chinese Herbs

The following Chinese herbs lend themselves to prepare as foods. Soups, stews and congees are the most frequent herbal preparations, done as follows:

1) The herbs may be prepared into teas first, then, the tea is used as all or part of the cooking water. This is especially useful for woody herbs like Huang Qi.

2) The herbs may be wrapped in a cotton cloth, cooked with the other ingredients and removed at the end. This is like the Chinese version of a "bouquet garni."

3) Herbs marked by * can be cooked loose and left in the soup to be eaten with the rest of the ingredients. Their textures are acceptable as foods.

There are many herbal wines that can be incorporated into foods. One popular one is SHOU WU CHIH, with the three main ingredients being He Shou Wu, Shu Di and Dang Gui. This wine is used to tonify Liver and Kidney and nourish Blood. It is a delicious addition to rice (add about 1-2 oz. per pot of rice.)

The **BASIC HERB SOUP** recipe is as follows:

1-3 ounces (30-90 grams) herb combination

½ -1½ lb. meat or fish (optional)

½ c. grain

¼ c. bean (optional)

1-3 c. chopped vegetables

6-8 c. water or broth

Cook herbs, meat, beans, grains and hard vegetables about 1 hour, until done. Add soft vegetables and short cooking herbs and finish cooking for 15-30 minutes. Season to taste with miso, tamari, soy sauce, rice vinegar or sea salt. The soup could be prepared in a crock pot on high for 3-4 hrs.

Cooking herbs for specific disharmonies:

WOOD DISHARMONIES:

1) LIVER QI STAGNATION: Fo Shou*, Qing Pi, Xiang Fu, Dill Seed*, Fennel Seed*, Coriander Seed*, Bo He

2) LIVER HEAT/FIRE: Pu Gong Ying*, Lu Dou*, Ju Hua*, Seaweeds*, Bo He

3) LIVER WIND: Gou Teng, Tian Ma*

4) LIVER BLOOD XU: Dang Gui*, Gou Qi Zi*, Gelatin*, He Shou Wu, Shu Di, Bai Shao

5) LIVER BLOOD STAGNATION: Dang Gui*, Chuan Xiong, Jiang Huang*, Hong Hua, Mu Er*, Saffron*

6) LIVER YIN XU: Gou Qi Zi*, Ju Hua*, Bai Shao, Sheng Di, Nu Zhen Zi

7) LIVER/GALL BLADDER DAMP HEAT: Yu Mi Xu, Yi Yi Ren*, Lu Dou*, Seaweeds*

FIRE DISHARMONIES:

1) HEART QI XU: Da Zao*, Ren Shen*, Long Yan Rou*, Fu Shen*, Lian Zi*

2) HEART YANG XU: Gui Zhi, Rou Gui*, Gan Jiang*, Xie Bai, Garlic*

3) HEART BLOOD XU: Suan Zao Ren*, Long Yan Rou*, Shu Di, Da Zao*, Bai Zi Ren, Dang Gui*, He Shou Wu

4) HEART YIN XU: Suan Zao Ren*, Sheng Di, Mai Men Dong, Bai He*

5) HEART BLOOD STAGNATION: Mu Er*, Dang Gui*, Dan Shen, Jiang Huang*, Hong Hua, Sheng Jiang*, Saffron*, Gui Zhi, Shan Zha, Chuan Xiong

6) HEART FIRE: Sheng Di, Lotus root*

7) PHLEGM MISTING HEART: HOT- Zhu Ru, Fu Shen*, Seaweeds; COLD- Yuan Zhi, Chen Pi, Fu Shen*

8) CALM SHEN: Suan Zao Ren*, Fu Shen*, Ling Zhi, Mu Li, Da Zao*, Basil*, Long Yan Rou*

EARTH DISHARMONIES:

1) SPLEEN QI XU: Huang Qi, Dang Shen*, Bai Zhu, Shan Yao*, Lian Zi*, Da Zao*, Fu Ling*, Ren Shen*
2) SPLEEN YANG XU: Gan Jiang*, Sheng Jiang*, Rou Gui*, all peppers*, all cardamons*, Garlic* + SP Qi Tonics
3) SPLEEN DAMP-COLD: Chen Pi*, Sheng Jiang*, Garlic*, Fu Ling*, Chi Xiao Dou*
4) SPLEEN DAMP-HEAT: Yi Yi Ren*, Lu Dou*, Chi Xiao Dou*, Fu Ling*, Yu Mi Xu
5) STOMACH FIRE: Seaweeds*, Lu Dou*, Shi Gao (short term)
6) STOMACH COLD: Sheng Jiang*, Gan Jiang*, Chen Pi*, Fennel*, Caraway*, Anise*seeds; Garlic*, all peppers*, all cardamons*
7) STOMACH YIN XU: Bai He*, Mai Men Dong, Shi Hu, Yu Zhu*
8) FOOD RETENTION: Mai Ya*, Gu Ya* (starches); Shan Zha (meats, fats); Ji Nei Jin* (all types of foods), Chen Pi*, Garlic*, Parsley*, all radishes*, Lemon*, Apple Cider Vinegar*

METAL DISHARMONIES:

1) LUNG QI XU: Gan Cao, Shan Yao*, Fu Ling*, Dang Shen*, Huang Qi, Tai Zi Shen*, Ren Shen*, Ling Zhi, Yi Tang*, Feng Mi*
2) LUNG YIN XU: Bai Mu Er*, Bai He*, Yu Zhu*, Mai Men Dong, Bei Sha Shen, Tian Men Dong, Xing Ren*, Feng Mi*, Yi Tang*, Chuan Bei Mu*
3) WIND COLD INVASION: Sheng Jiang*, Zi Su Ye*, Cong Bai*, Gui Zhi, Cilantro*
4) WIND HEAT INVASION: Bo He, Sang Ye, Ju Hua*, Niu Bang Zi, Niu Bang Gen*, Dan Dou Chi*, Cilantro*
5) WIND DRYNESS INVASION: Bai Mu Er*, Sang Ye, Ju Hua*, Chuan Bei Mu*, Xing Ren*, Bai He*, Feng Mi*, Yi Tang*
6) HOT PHLEGM: Jie Geng*, Lai Fu Zi*, Chuan Bei Mu*, Seaweeds*, Zhu Ru
7) COLD PHLEGM: Chen Pi*, Jie Geng*, Lai Fu Zi*, Bai Jie Zi*

8) LARGE INTESTINE DAMP HEAT: Jin Yin Hua, Yu Mi Xu, Lu Dou*, Yi Yi Ren*, Pu Gong Ying*

9) LARGE INTESTINE DRYNESS: Bai Mu Er*, Hei Zi Ma*, Tao Ren*, Xing Ren*, Ya Ma Ren (flax seed)*

WATER DISHARMONIES:

1) KIDNEY YANG XU: Hu Lu Ba*, Du Zhong, Dong Chong Xia Cao*, Rou Gui*, Gan Jiang*, Shan Zhu Yu*, Garlic*

2) KIDNEY YIN XU: Tian Men Dong, Gou Qi Zi*, Nu Zhen Zi, He Shou Wu, Shu Di, Sheng Di, Seaweeds*

3) KIDNEY JING XU: Gou Qi Zi*, He Shou Wu, Shu Di, Tu Si Zi, Lian Zi*

4) KIDNEY/BLADDER QI XU: Lian Zi*, Qian Shi*, Fu Pen Zi*, Shan Zhu Yu*, Rou Dou Kou*

5) KIDNEY UNABLE TO GRASP LUNG QI: Ren Shen*, Hu Tao Ren*, He Tao Ren*, Dong Chong Xia Cao*, Shan Yao*

6) DAMP-HEAT IN BLADDER: Jin Yin Hua, Fu Ling*, Yu Mi Xu, Pu Gong Ying*, Yi Yi Ren*, Chi Xiao Dou*

Herbal Recipes:

Congees

A congee, also known as jook, porridge or gruel, is a soupy grain dish, typically eaten for breakfast, but may be used for other meals by patients who are weak or chronically ill. Congees are highly digestible and assimilable and good for patients with weak digestion, fatigue, poor appetite or those convalescing from surgery or illness.

They are traditionally cooked using rice or millet as the grain, but other grains will also work such as barley, cornmeal, quinoa or a combination of grains. The basic recipe can be modified with the addition of therapeutic foods, medicinal herbs and spices.

Basic Congee Recipe

1 c. rice (white, brown, sweet, basmati)

5-10 c. water (depending on how thick or thin you want the dish to be)

Cook for about 4-6 hours on a low flame or overnight in a crock pot. The finished congee could be mildly seasoned to taste with sea salt, miso or honey.

The following additions would be added at the beginning of the cooking process:

1. ¼ c. mung beans to clear heat and toxins
2. ¼ c. aduki beans, ¼ c. Yi Yi Ren (Coix) to promote urination, reduce damp and heat
3. 2 chopped celery stalks to clear heat, reduce hypertension
4. 1 chopped carrot to promote digestion and strengthen the Lung
5. 1 t. Fennel seeds or Coriander seed to relieve gas and bloating
6. 5 pitted Da Zao (Chinese dates) and 3 slices fresh Ginger to harmonize the Stomach and relieve nausea or vomiting
7. ¼ c. Gou Qi Zi (Lycii berries) to benefit the eyes and nourish Blood and Yin
8. 10 grams Huang Qi (Astragalus), 10 grams Shan Yao (Chinese Yam) and 5 Shitake mushrooms to benefit the immune system (remove the Huang Qi at the end of cooking-it will stay woody)
9. ¼ c. dried seaweed such as wakame, nori or dulse to reduce yellow phlegm
10. 2 t. Turmeric powder to activate the blood and relieve pain
11. ½ c. chopped walnuts, almonds, pine nuts or sesame seed to promote a bowel movement
12. 1 chopped pear, ¼ c. chopped almonds to descend the Lung Qi and stop cough

The following additions would be added at the end of the cooking, the last 10-15 minutes:

1. ¼ c. chopped Mint to promote sweat and relieve fever and sore throat
2. ¼ c. chopped Parsley to promote digestion and relieve food stagnation, bloating and indigestion
3. ¼ c. chopped scallions and 6 slices of fresh Ginger to relieve chills and nasal congestion

Herbal Pumpkin Mushroom Soup

Cook 1 large pumpkin (or sub 1 large can pumpkin puree) until soft; remove peel, then blend with the cooking water (about 6-8 cups).

In a separate pan, simmer the following herbs with enough water to cover, until soft (about 30 minutes):
10 g. Dioscorea yam (Shan Yao)
10 g. Codonopsis (Dang Shen)
5 g. Lycii berries (Gou Qi Zi)
5 g. Longan fruit (Long Yan Rou)
1 small handful Dulse seaweed

Saute in olive oil until soft:
15 fresh Shitake mushrooms, thinly sliced
1 small sweet onion, chopped
1 red bell pepper, chopped

Combine all of the above ingredients with the pumpkin puree. Season to taste with miso, Bragg's Liquid Amino Seasoning (or substitute tamari soy sauce), ginger juice, coriander powder and turmeric powder. Garnish with chopped cilantro and/or chives.

TCM Properties: Tonify and Regulate Qi and Blood / Calm the Spirit

Dang Gui Cornish Hen Soup

1 Cornish hen
¼ c. rice
2 parsnips, chopped
2 stalks celery, chopped
2 carrots, chopped
1 small onion, chopped
2 leaves of kale, chopped
15 g. Dang Gui
10 Da Zao (dates), seed removed
5 slices Sheng Jiang (ginger)
1 handful wakame seaweed
Cook together with 8 c. water until hen is cooked (about 45-60 minutes), then remove the bones and chop the meat. Season to taste with miso.

TCM Properties: Tonify Qi and Blood, Move Blood, Harmonize Middle Burner

Autumn Pear Syrup (Dr. Maoshing Ni's)

3 fresh Asian pears, diced
10 g. Kuan Dong Hua (Farfara Flower)
12 g. Bai He (Lily Bulb)
12 g. Mai Men Dong (Ophiopoginis Root)
10 g. Chuan Bei Mu (Fritillaria bulb)
1 c. honey

Cook the herbs and the pears in 6 c. of water over a low flame for about 1 ½ hours. Strain and then concentrate the liquid by slowly cooking it down to about 1 c. Slowly stir in the honey over a very small flame, continue to stir until it almost boils. Remove from flame and let it cool into a syrup, then refrigerate. Take 1 Tbsp. dissolved in hot water 3-4 times a day for at least 2 weeks.

TCM Properties: Moisten Lung, Stops Cough

Happy Liver Rice

1 c. rice (basmati or jasmine is best to move Qi and dampness)

¼ c. mung bean (Lu Dou)

10 g. Fo Shou (Citron)

1 small fennel bulb, diced

10 g. Bai He (Lily bulbs)

Cook until water is absorbed. Season to taste with salt.

TCM Properties: Regulate Liver Qi, Tonify Spleen Qi, Calm Shen

Herbal Eggs

2 eggs

20 g. Sang Ji Sheng*

4 c. water

Cook eggs until hard boiled (about 10 minutes). Peel eggs and return to pan to continue to cook with the herbs for another 10 minutes. Strain tea. Eat eggs and drink tea.

TCM Properties: Tonify Qi, Blood and Yin; Secure the Fetus.
* substitute Yi Mu Cao (Motherwort) to move blood, regulates menses, relieve dysmenorrhea
* substitute Ai Ye (Chinese Mugwort) to warms the uterus, relieve dysmenorrheal

Salmon Stew

½ - 1 lb. Wild Salmon, skinned and cubed

¼ c. rice

1 small sweet potato, cubed

2 stalks celery, chopped

1 small onion, chopped

2 leaves kale, chopped

10 g. Dang Gui

10 g. Dang Shen (Codonopsis)

5 Da Zao (dates), seeds removed

5 slices fresh ginger

1 handful wakame seaweed

1 clove garlic, chopped

Cook all ingredients in 8 c. water for 1 hour. Season to taste with miso.

TCM Properties: Tonify Qi and Blood, Harmonize Middle Burner

Drain The Damp Fish Soup

½ -1 lb. Tilapia or other white fish, cubed

¼ c. Yi Yi Ren (Coix)

¼ c. Aduki beans, presoaked

10 g. Fu Ling (Poria), crushed finely

5 stalks celery, chopped

3 slices fresh Ginger

1 handful dulse

1 handful of Parsley, chopped finely

Cook all ingredients except the parsley with 8 c. water for 1 hour. When done, add the parsley and season to taste with Bragg's Liquid Aminos or a little sea salt.

TCM Properties: Tonify Spleen Qi, Promote Urination, Drain Dampness.

Sun Cycles: Eating with the Seasons

Imagine your energy is like that of a tree - if you observe the natural flow of the tree's Qi through the seasons, you get an idea of being in harmony with Nature. In the Winter the energy is deep in the trunk and roots, storing up for seasons to come. In Spring the tree's Qi moves upward and outward to the branches, forming buds. By Summer the energy is at its peak of expression in the leaves, flowers and forming fruits. Late Summer the fruits have formed and are becoming ripened, reflecting the tree's strongest Qi. Contained in those fruits are the seeds for creating a whole new generation of trees - that is powerful Qi! Autumn causes the tree's energy to recede into the large branches and trunk, causing the leaves, unsupported by Qi, to fall. Then by Winter time, the Qi has again penetrated to deep in the trunk and roots.

When our energy goes dramatically counter to this natural flow, we encounter health problems. For example, the excessive party behavior from November through January expends our Qi, the opposite of storage - the net effect is high incidence of depression, anxiety and weakened immune systems. In Springtime if we are still indulging in the heavier Winter storage fare, eating lots of meat, cheese and rich dishes, the end result is stagnant Liver Qi, allergies, headaches, skin conditions and lots of phlegm. A visit to the local farmers' market will get you in touch with the fruits and vegetables that are truly in season for your locale.

Guidelines for Each Season:

LATE SUMMER –

This is the transition season between the warmth of Spring and Summer and the coolness Fall and Winter, associated with the Earth element, our digestive system. Dampness may present easily now, so the diet must be "Spleen-friendly" - complex carbohydrates, whole grains, legumes, plenty of vegetables, some animal protein and limit the dampening foods like fruit juices, salads and refined sweets.

Herbs to strengthen Spleen and Stomach: Codonopsis (Dang Shen), Poria (Fu Ling), Dioscorea (Shan Yao), Licorice (Gan Cao).

Herbs to facilitate digestion: Hawthorn (Shan Zha), Citrus Peel (Chen Pi), Ginger (Sheng Jiang), Cardamom (all types), cooking herbs that are seeds - Fennel, Anise, Caraway, Coriander, Cumin

Earth Disharmonies:

SPLEEN QI DEFICIENCY
Adequate protein: animal products, unrefined grains and beans, nuts and seeds
Sweet vegetables like carrots, beets, sweet potato, winter squash, parsnips
String beans, peas, Shitake mushrooms
Cherries, dates, raisins, honey, molasses
Limit - refined grains, sugar, cold raw foods

SPLEEN YANG DEFICIENCY
Use the SPLEEN QI DEFICIENCY FOODS plus warming spices like Ginger, Garlic, Pepper, Cinnamon, Nutmeg, Cardamom, Fennel seeds
Quinoa, pan-roasted oats, lamb, beef, chicken, turkey, shrimp, baked root vegetables
> *Limit - refined grains, sugar, fruit juice, cold raw foods, citrus, melons, tomatoes, soy foods*

DAMPNESS DISTRESSING THE SPLEEN
> DAMP HEAT – bitter greens, celery, mung beans, Yi Yi Ren, barley, aduki beans, kidney beans, millet, amaranth, rye, rice (especially basmati), pumpkin, mushrooms, pumpkin, fish
> *Limit - refined grains, sugar, spicy foods, oily foods, coffee, alcohol*

> DAMP COLD – mustard greens, turnip, Garlic, rice (especially basmati), Ginger, fish, beef

Limit - refined grains, sugar, citrus, melons, bananas, tomatoes, soy foods, oily foods, dairy products, cold raw foods

FOOD STAGNATION
Parsley, radish, apple, lemon, Hawthorn Berry (Shan Zha), sprouted rice or barley, chicken gizzard, vinegar, Garlic, papaya, pineapple, mango
Limit - large meals, late night eating, sugar, refined grains

STOMACH HEAT
Bitter greens, bitter melon, soy products, potato, watermelon, pear, banana, Napa cabbage, celery, seaweed, mung bean, lotus root
Limit - spicy foods, coffee, alcohol, fried foods, acidy fruits

AUTUMN –

The energy is moving inward. Begin to eat more warming foods, root vegetables, mostly cooked foods and try to reduce the cooling foods such as fruit juices and salads. Seasonal fruits such as apples and pears may be prepared with warming spices like ginger and cinnamon. For those who tend towards dryness during this time may benefit from raw pears and pear juice. This is the time to reinforce and moisten (if needed) the Lung and Large Intestine. This is a time to "let go" of the past. Grief often is expressed now.

Foods to tonify and moisten Lung: Oily fish such as Salmon, Pear, Flaxseed, Loquat, Papaya, Carrot, Sweet Potato, Soymilk, Pinenuts, Almonds
Herbs to Tonify Lung Qi: Astragalus (Huang Qi), Codonopsis (Dang Shen), Ophiopogon (Mai Men Dong), Dioscorea (Shan Yao), Lily Bulb (Bai He)

Spices/Herbs/foods for reducing phlegm in the Lung: Garlic, Ginger (Sheng Jiang), Cayenne, Citrus peel (Chen Pi), Onions
Metal Disharmonies:

LUNG QI DEFICIENCY
Whole grains – rice, oats, barley

Beans, especially the white ones like lima, navy, soy
Animal proteins – fish, chicken, turkey, goat's milk, eggs
Sweet fruits like cherries, persimmons, pears, papaya, strawberries, loquat, tangerine
Almonds, walnuts, peanuts
Limit - refined grains, sugar, cold raw foods, dairy products if there is phlegm

LUNG YIN DEFICIENCY
Seaweeds, oily fish, duck, potato, pear, dairy products, eggs, white wood ears (Bai Mu Er), almonds, peanuts, soy products
> *Limit – spicy foods, coffee, alcohol*

LUNG HEAT
Bitter flavored foods, seaweed, Napa cabbage, pear, peach, loquat, lemon, papaya, strawberries, carrots, burdock root, lotus root
Limit - spicy foods, coffee, alcohol

PHLEGM IN THE LUNG
See HEART PHLEGM FOODS

EXTERNAL WIND ATTACKING THE LUNG
WIND – COLD – scallions, Ginger, mustard greens, carrots, cabbage, Basil, parsnips
> WIND – HEAT – Mint, summer squash, carrots, Napa cabbage, Burdock
> Root, celery, Asian pears
Limit - heavy foods, refined grains, sugar, coffee, alcohol

WINTER –

This is the time for storage. We should be conserving our energy and replenishing our reserves. Weak Kidney energy may present with a worsening of fears during this time of year. Exhaustion now is particularly harmful, and may continue to be felt in the year to come. This is the time to be sure to get to bed early. Diet should focus on warming and strengthening Qi, Yang and Blood. This will also be the time to eat a little more salty flavored foods such as seaweed, miso and tamari for strengthening the Kidney.

Warming/tonifying foods for winter: lamb, beef, chicken, turkey, salmon, walnuts, chestnuts, black beans, black sesame seeds, oats, quinoa, parsnips, cherries, dried fruits stewed with warming spices, winter squash

Winter herbs: Ginseng (Ren Shen), Astragalus (Huang Qi), Ginger (Gan Jiang), Cinnamon (Rou Gui), Cloves (Ding Xiang), Parsley, Cardamom, Dang Gui, Dioscorea (Shan Yao)

Water Disharmonies:

KIDNEY YIN DEFICIENCY
Sweet, watery vegetables, seaweeds
Black beans, soybeans, wheat
Black sesame seeds, flax seeds
Dairy products, eggs, oily fish, pork, clam, duck, oyster
Sweet, dark-colored fruits like cherries, berries, grapes
Limit - spicy foods, coffee, alcohol

KIDNEY YANG DEFICIENCY
Beef, chicken, turkey, lamb, trout, salmon, shrimp
Onion family – Garlic, chives, leeks
Pungent spices like Ginger, Cinnamon, Cloves
Black beans, walnuts, cherries, string beans, chestnuts, parsnip
Limit - cold raw foods, sugar

KIDNEY QI DEFICIENCY
Sour flavored foods like raspberries, blackberries, Rosehips, leeks
Dark colored foods like black beans, kidney beans, black sesame seeds
Wheat, wild rice, black rice
Limit - cold raw foods, sugar

KIDNEY JING DEFICIENCY

Oyster, mussel, anchovy, chicken, clams, fertile eggs, dairy products, royal jelly (from bees), Cordyceps (Dong Chong Xia Cao), microalgae (Spirulina, Chlorella), Lycii berries (Gou Qi Zi), black sesame seeds
Limit - cold raw foods, sugar, refined foods, coffee, alcohol

DAMP – HEAT IN THE BLADDER

Bitter foods like endive, romaine, bitter melon, asparagus, artichoke, Dandelion greens
Cranberries, blueberries, watermelon, lemon, aduki beans, mung beans, Yi Yi Ren, barley
Limit - sugar, spicy foods, fried foods, coffee, alcohol

SPRING –

Diet should nourish the Liver and help it to dispel and disperse stagnation.

Dark leafy greens, sprouts, celery, spinach and green tea to cleanse the Liver and the blood and relieve stagnation
Lemon juice to clear the Liver; Flax seed, sunflower seeds to nourish the Liver
Light meats, legumes, whole grains and fruits.

Movement!! Nothing will move your stagnation like exercise. Regulate sleep, with a goal of being asleep before the Wood hours begin at 11. No late night eating or overeating.

Moving/cleansing Liver herbs: Dandelion (Pu Gong Ying), Milk Thistle Seed, Turmeric (Jiang Huang), Burdock root (Niu Bang Gen), Fennel seed (Xiao Hui Xiang), Citron (Fo Shou) and Green Tangerine peel (Qing Pi)
Pungent herbs to reduce the leftover dampness of winter: Cayenne, Garlic, Paprika

Nourishing Liver herbs: Lycii berries (Gou Qi Zi), White peony root (Bai Shao), Dang Gui, Ziziphus seed (Suan Zao Ren)

Wood Disharmonies:

LIVER QI STAGNATION FOODS

Onion family - onion, Garlic, leeks

Cabbage family - cabbage, broccoli, Brussels sprouts, mustard greens, turnip, kale

Pungent foods, herbs and spices – radish, Basil, Cilantro, Arugula, Coriander seed, Fennel seed, Turmeric, Cayenne, Cardamom, Mint

Fibrous foods - celery, whole grains, beans

Sour flavored foods – lemon, grapefruit, vinegar, plums, green apples

> *Limit – refined grains, sugar, fried foods, chemical additives, low fiber diets*

LIVER HEAT FOODS

Bitter foods – celery, romaine, endive, Dandelion greens, asparagus, rye, amaranth

Mung beans (and sprouts), soybeans (and products), seaweeds, cucumber, summer squash, tomatoes, sunflower sprouts, artichoke, Burdock root, lemon, grapefruit, bitter melon, celery

Limit – spicy foods, alcohol coffee, lamb, beef, trout

LIVER BLOOD AND YIN NOURISHING FOODS

Nuts and seeds – especially flax and black sesame

Chlorophyll-rich foods (green vegetables and seaweeds)

Sweet fruits - especially berries, cherries, grapes, avocado, dates, figs, apricots, mulberries, Lycii berries

Sweet vegetables like beets, carrots, potatoes, parsnips, sweet potato; molasses

Black beans, soybeans, oats, black sesame seeds

Dairy products, eggs, chicken, pork (for Yin), beef (for Blood), oily fish (like salmon)

Limit – spicy foods, alcohol, coffee

LIVER YANG ASCENDING

Asparagus, apples, barley, celery, sunflower seeds, barley, tomatoes, eggplant, wheat, peas, bitter flavored foods

Limit – spicy foods, alcohol, coffee

LIVER WIND

Celery, oats, black beans, black sesame seeds, bitter greens

Limit – shellfish (especially shrimp, crab, prawns and lobster), eggs, dairy products, greasy foods

LIVER – GALL BLADDER DAMP - HEAT

Bitter flavored foods, barley, Yi Yi Ren, mung beans, aduki beans, rye, pumpkin, celery, bitter melon, bamboo shoots, radishes, olives, seaweed, apples, pears, grapefruit, lemon

Limit – refined grains, sugar, fried foods, spicy foods, coffee, alcohol

LIVER BLOOD STAGNATION

Pungent flavored foods like onion, Garlic, Scallion, Ginger, vinegar, Turmeric and Saffron

Eggplant, black wood ear mushroom, Shitake mushroom

Hawthorn berry (Shan Zha), cayenne pepper, chili pepper

Limit – cold foods, refined foods

SUMMER –

Foods should be light and easy to digest such as fruits, salads, grains and legumes. We will need to guard against getting overheated and overcooled. Both too much spicy foods and too much cold foods can lead to Summer time health problems. The goal is to stay cool, dispel heat from the Heart and replenish fluids.

Some bitter flavored greens can strengthen the heart and eliminate excess fluids and heat.

Foods/herbs to prevent and treat Summer heat: Mung Bean (Lu Dou), watermelon, cucumber, summer squash, tomato, lemon, soybean sprouts, Honeysuckle flowers (Jin Yin Hua). Some spicy flavored herbs such as curry and peppers can open the pores, promote perspiration and cool the body. Keep both bitter and spicy to a minimum - small amounts are balancing, large amounts will cause problems.

Herbs to drink as refreshing summer beverages: Peppermint (Bo He), Hibiscus, Chrysanthemum (Ju Hua), Lemon Balm and Green Tea.

Fire Disharmonies:

HEART YIN AND BLOOD DEFICIENCY
See Liver Yin and Blood foods

HEART QI DEFICIENCY
See Spleen Qi deficiency foods

HEART YANG DEFICIENCY
Use Heart Qi deficiency foods plus warming spices like: Cinnamon, Ginger, Clove, Nutmeg, Cumin, Cardamom
Raspberries, cherries, shrimp, walnuts, lamb, chestnuts, trout, salmon
Limit – cold foods, raw foods

HEART BLOOD STAGNATION
See Liver Blood stagnation

HEART PHELGM CONDITIONS:
HOT PHLEGM – pears, apples, daikon radish, seaweed, bitter greens, bamboo shoots, raw almonds, button mushrooms, basmati rice

Limit - refined grains, sugar, dairy products, alcohol, coffee
COLD PHLEGM – roasted almonds, walnuts, Ginger, Garlic, mustard greens and seed, pepper, scallions, Cinnamon, pepper, basmati rice
Limit - refined grains, sugar, dairy products, alcohol, raw foods

HEART SHEN DISTURBANCES:
Whole grains – especially brown rice, oats, barley
Chlorophyll-rich green vegetables like lettuce, kale, basil, holy basil
Mineral rich foods like whole fish, seaweeds, celery
Limit – sugar, refined foods, spicy foods, coffee, alcohol

Moon Cycles: Harmonizing for Women

Females Have Special Needs:

Pregnancy – more protein (Qi/Blood tonics); not too dampening; appropriately moving, avoiding strongly moving foods
Post-partum – replenish what was lost (Qi, Blood, Jing)
Lactation – more Blood tonics and fluids
Pre-menstrual – regulate Qi and Blood; avoid overly cooling
Post-menses – replenish Blood, Liver, Kidney
Peri- and post- menopausal – declining Kidney Jing (+Yin/Yang)

For brilliant charts, diagrams and information on the phases of the female menstrual cycle and reproductive system, refer to the following text book:
Obstetrics and Gynecology in Chinese Medicine by Giovanni Maciocia, 1998

Appendix 2

Common Food Plant Families

GRAINS:

Gramineae or Poaceae (Grass family) - all cereal grains belong to this family, as does sugarcane. Amaranth, Quinoa, and Buckwheat are not in this family. The gluten containing ones are wheat, spelt, kamut, rye, and barley. Oats do not contain gluten, but are often processed in factories that also process gluten grains, so look for guaranteed gluten-free oats. Corn is usually genetically modified.

Rice, Corn, Wheat, Barley, Rye, Oats, Spelt, Kamut, Millet

BEANS:

Leguminosae or Fabaceae (Legume family) - all beans (legumes) belong to this family, as well as peanuts. Beans are nutrient dense and loaded with fiber. Larger beans are more difficult to digest. Soybeans can be a digestive challenge for many and are usually genetically modified. Phyto-estrogen components are found in some of the members, most notably in Soybeans and Red Clover blossoms.

Soy, Lima, Black, Pinto, White Northern, Fava, Aduki, Mung, Lentil, Peas, Garbonzos
(Chick Peas), Peanuts, Alfalfa, Red Clover

VEGETABLES:

Liliaceae (Lily family – includes the sub-family Alliums/Onion family) – these improve circulation and are highly anti-microbial for many pathogens. Garlic is the hottest and cautioned with hot dry eyes and mouth sores.
Onion, Garlic, Chive, Shallot, Leek, Asparagus

Cruciferae or Brassicaceae (Cabbage family) – known for their rich assortment of anti-cancer, anti-oxidant components. This family can inhibit thyroid hormone production, especially raw, but cooked cabbage family foods should also be eaten minimally by hypothyroid patients.
Broccoli, Cabbage, Cauliflower, Kale, Kohlrabi, Mustard, Turnip, Rutabaga, Radish, Watercress, Arugula, Radish, Watercress, Brussel Sprouts

Solanaceae (Nightshade family) - members contain the alkaloid solanine, which is reduced if cooked. The foods in this family can contribute to worsening joint pain in sensitive patients. Several members are poisonous, such as belladona, henbane and nightshade. Tobacco is another member.
Tomato, Potato, Peppers (bell, cayenne, jalapeno, etc.), Eggplant, Tomatillos, Lycii berries (Gou Qi Zi/Gou Ji berries)

Chenopodiaceae (Goosefoot family) - some members contain oxalic acid, which is reduced if cooked. Beet greens, spinach and chard should be limited in patients with a history of kidney stones (commonly composed of calcium oxalate).
Beet, Spinach, Chard, Amaranth, Quinoa, Epazote

Compositae or Asteraceae (Sunflower family) – many of these are beneficial for the liver, gall bladder and blood sugar issues. Many medicinal herbs are in this family which reduce toxins.
Artichoke, Jerusalem Artichoke, Lettuces, Sunflower, Dandelion, Tarragon, Mugwort, Calendula, Chrysanthemum, Echinacea, Burdock, Yarrow, Milk Thistle, Stevia

Umbelliferae or Apiaceae (Carrot family) – these members are high in minerals. Some of the umbel seeds such as Coriander, Fennel, Celery, Caraway, and Anise, are made into tea to relieve digestive complaints and colic. Many herbs in this family are pain relieving. Several members are poisonous such as poison hemlock and water hemlock.
Carrot, Celery, Parsley, Parsnip, Cilantro, Fennel, Dill, Lovage, Asafoetida, Angelicas

Cucurbitaceae (Gourd family) – this family assists in normalizing fluids.
Cucumber, Summer squash, Winter squash, Pumpkin, Bitter melon, Luffa

Convolvulaceae (Morning glory family) – the many varieties of sweet potatoes that grow around the world are important foods that provide healthy carbohydrates, beta-carotene, and fiber.
Sweet Potatoes – come in many colors including yellow, orange, white and purple. Supermarkets sell mislabeled "yams" that are botanically a variety of sweet potato. Whether they are the moist orange flesh or the firmer yellow flesh, both are sweet potatoes.
Do not ever eat morning glory seeds, which are toxic and hallucinogenic.

Discordance (Yam family) - Yams provide healthy carbohydrates, hormone support, and strengthen digestion. Wear gloves when peeling these because the raw yam can irritate the skin. The only one that is safely eaten raw is the Chinese Yam.
Chinese Yam (Dioscorea opposita/Shan Yao) – these would be found in a specialty grocery.
Mexican Wild Yam (Dioscorea paniculata) – used as a source of phyto-hormones

Polygonaceae (Knotweed family) – mostly herbs and ornamentals are in this family.
Buckwheat, Rhubarb, Sorrel, Knotweed, He Shou Wu (Fo Ti)

Labiatae or Lamiaceae (Mint family) – this family is known for its aromatic oils contained in the leaves, stems and flowers. Short cooking time will preserve those oils. Many cooking and medicinal herbs are in this family.

All Mints, Rosemary, Lavender, Sage, Basil, Marjoram, Thyme, Savory, Catnip, Scullcap, Prunella, Motherwort, Lemon Balm

Zingiberaceae (Ginger family) – important medicinal food and spice family with both Ginger and Turmeric as members. Many of the herb members are qi and blood activating to relieve pain, reduce swelling, anti-pathogenic, and rich in aromatic oils that improve digestion. This family includes plants for making dyes and perfumes, as well as ornamentals, cultivated for their showy flowers.

Ginger, Turmeric, Cardamom, Galangal

FRUITS AND NUTS:

Rosaceae (Rose family) – the seeds of some of these contain a cyanide compound and should not be ingested by pets, or people in large amounts, especially apple, peach and apricot pits.

Apple, Cherry, Pear, Peach, Plum, Apricot, Blackberry, Raspberry, Strawberry, Hawthorn, Loquat, Almond, Quince

Ericacea (Heath family) – several members benefit the urinary and cardio-vascular systems. The berries are very high in antioxidants and low in sugar. Uva Ursi (Bearberry) and Manzanita are herb members for the bladder. Bilberry improves circulation to the eyes and is used for degenerative eye disorders.

Cranberry, Blueberry, Bilberry, Huckleberry

Moraceae (Mulberry family) – these fruits are mucilaginous, moistening, and tonifying.

Mulberry, Fig, Breadfruit

Rutaceae (Citrus family) – all of the dried citrus peels can be used in teas for phlegm conditions
Orange, Tangerine, Lemon, Lime, Grapefruit, Citron, Kumquat

Cucurbitaceae (Gourd family) – useful in summertime to rehydrate and move fluids
Watermelon, Cantaloupe, all melon varieties

Anacardiacea (Mango family) – wear gloves when peeling mangoes because the latex exuded from the peel can cause an allergic reaction on the skin. Poison oak and poison ivy are also in this family.
Mango, Cashew, Pistachio

Juglandaceae (Walnut family) – the members contain large amounts of arginine which can stimulate an outbreak of herpes.
Walnuts, Pecans, Hickory Nuts

SEAWEEDS AND OTHER ALGAE:
Algae are classified botanically by color and size. These foods are all mineral rich.

Macro-algae (Seaweeds) - all are cooling; Dulse and Nori are the least cooling. These are not appropriate for someone with an iodine allergy or autoimmune thyroid conditions.
Kombu (Kun Bu), Wakame, Hiziki, Arame, Dulse, Nori

Micro-algae - all are cooling; Chlorella is least cooling. All are nutrient dense, chlorophyl rich, and a protein source for vegans and vegetarians.
Spirulina, Chlorella, Blue-green algae

MEDICINAL MUSHROOMS:
Mushrooms are all members of the **Fungi Kingdom** of organisms – all of the mushrooms benefits fluid imbalances in our bodies, including damp-heat

conditions. Many also benefit the immune system and increase vitality. Many varieties are used with cancer patients to support their immune systems and protect them from injury by chemotherapy and radiation. These are commonly consumed as foods.

Shitake (Xiang Gu) – strengthen the immune system; control cholesterol; anti-cancer.

Maitake – strengthen the immune system; anti-cancer.

White wood ears (Bai Mu Er) – nourish the yin of the stomach and lungs, treating dry cough or stool.

Black wood ears (Hei Mu Er) – move the blood to relieve pain; contraindicated with blood thinners or with bleeding conditions.

Enoki – especially good for the lungs; anti-viral; cancer protection; reduce allergies.

White button (Portebellos are a version of this one) – clear heat and dampness.

Ling Zhi (Ganoderma/Reishi) – balances both over active and under active immune system

Chaga (Inonotus obliquus) – anti-cancer, anti-viral. This makes a delicious tea.

Cordyceps (Dong Chong Xia Cao) – supports immunity by strengthening lungs, liver and kidneys. It is traditionally cooked into soups with duck, chicken, pork or fish.

For more information about the medicinal mushrooms:
Medicinal Mushrooms by Christopher Hobbs
Medicinal Mushrooms: A Clinical Guide by Martin Powell
Healing Mushrooms by George M. Halpern

Suggested Reading

Traditional Chinese Medicine

Beinfield, Harriet and Efrem Korngold. *Between Heaven and Earth: A Guide to Chinese Medicine*. New York: Random House Publishing (Ballantine Books), 1991.

Flaws, Bob and Philippe Sionneau. *The Treatment of Modern Western Medical Diseases with Chinese* Medicine (2nd Ed). Boulder, CO: Blue Poppy Press, 2005.

Kaptchuk, Ted J. *The Web That Has No Weaver.* New York: McGraw-Hill, 2000.

Liang, Lifang. *Contemporary Gynecology*. Boulder, CO: Blue Poppy Press, 2010.

L'Orange, Darlena with Gary Dolowich. *Ancient Roots, Many Branches*. Twin Lakes, WI: Lotus Press, 2002.

Maciocia, Giovanni. *Clinical Pearls*. Santa Barbara, CA: Su Wen Press, 2013.

Maciocia, Giovanni. *The Foundations of Chinese Medicine (2nd Ed)*. New York: Elsevier (Churchill Livingstone), 2005.

Maciocia, Giovanni. *The Practice of Chinese Medicine (2nd Ed)*. New York: Elsevier (Churchill Livingstone), 2008.

Maciocia, Giovanni. *The Psyche in Chinese Medicine.* New York: Elsevier (Churchill Livingstone), 2009.

Ni, Maoshing. *The Yellow Emperor's Classic of Medicine.* Boston: Shambhala, 1995.

Ni, Yitian. *Navigating the Channels of Traditional Chinese Medicine.* San Diego, CA: Complementary Medicine Press, 1996.

Nutrition

Acquista, Angelo. *The Mediterranean Prescription.* New York: Ballantine Books, 2006.

Bratman, Steven with David Knight. *Health Food Junkies.* New York: Broadway Books, 2000.

Campbell, T. Colin and Thomas M. Campbell II, *The China Study.* Dallas, TX: BenBella Books, 2006.

Colbin, Annemarie. *Food and Healing.* New York: Ballantine Books, 1986.

Colbin, Annemarie. *The Whole-Food Guide to Strong Bones.* Oakland, CA: New Harbinger Publications, 2009.

Haas, Elson. *Staying Healthy With the Seasons.* Berkeley, CA: Celestial Arts, 2003.

Kastner, Joerg. *Chinese Nutrition Therapy: Dietetics in Traditional Chinese Medicine.* New York: Thieme, 2004.

Lu, Henry C. *Chinese Natural Cures.* New York: Black Dog and Leventhal Publishers, 2005.

Murray, Michael. *The Healing Power of Foods.* Rocklin, CA: Prima Publishing, 1993.

Ni, Daoshing. *Sitting Moon: A Guide to Rejuvenation after Pregnancy*. Los Angeles: The Tao of Wellness Press, 2010.

Ni, Maoshing and Cathy McNease. *The Tao of Nutrition (3rd Ed)*. Los Angeles: Tao of Wellness Press, 2009.

Perlmutter, David. *Grain Brain*. New York: Little, Brown, and Co, 2013.

Pitchford, Paul. *Healing with Whole Foods: Asian Traditions and Modern Nutrition*. Berkeley, CA: North Atlantic Books, 2002.

Pollan, Michael. *In Defense of Food*. New York: The Penguin Press, 2008.

Shomon, Mary J. *Living Well with Autoimmune Disease*. New York: Harper Collins, 2002.

Herbs
Bensky, Dan, Steven Clavey, & Erich Stoger, *Chinese Herbal Medicine: Materia Medica (3rd Ed)*. Seattle: Eastland Press, 2004.

Chen, John K. and Tina T. Chen. *Chinese Herbal Formulas and Applications*. City of Industry, CA: Art of Medicine Press, 2009.

Chen, John K. and Tina T. Chen. *Chinese Medical Herboloty and Pharmacology*. City of Industry, CA: Art of Medicine Press, 2004.

Fratkin, Jake Paul. *Essential Chinese Formulas*. Boulder, CO: Shya Publications, 2014.

Gladstar, Rosemary. *Herbal Healing for Women*. New York: Simone and Schuster, 1993.

Han, Henry, Glenn E. Miller, and Nancy Deville. *Ancient Herbs, Modern Medicine*. New York: Bantam, 2003.

Harrar, Sari and Sara Altshul O'Donnell. *Woman's Book of Healing Herbs.* Emmaus, PA: Rodale Press, 1999.

Hobbs, Christopher and Leslie Gardner. *Grow It, Heal It.* New York: Rodale, 2013.

Hobbs, Christopher. *Medicinal Mushrooms.* Santa Cruz, CA: Botanica Press, 1995.

Holmes, Peter with Jing Wang. *The Traditional Chinese Medicine Materia Medica Clinical Reference and Study Guide.* Boulder, CO: Snow Lotus Press, 2002.

Johnson, Rebecca, Steven Foster, Tieraona Low Dog, and David Kiefer. *The National Geographic Guide to Medicinal Herbs.* Washington, DC: National Geographic Society, 2010.

L'Orange, Darlena. *Herbal Healing Secrets of the Orient.* Paramus, NJ: Prentice Hall, 1998.

Mars, Brigitte. *Natural First Aid.* Pownal, VT: Storey Books. 1999.

Ni, Maoshing. *Chinese Herbology Made Easy.* Los Angeles: 7 Star Communications, 2003.

Schafer, Peg. *The Chinese Medicinal Herb Farm.* White River Junction, VT: Chelsea Green Publishing, 2011.

Teeguarden, Ron. *The Ancient Wisdom of the Chinese Tonic Herbs.* New York: Grand Central Publishing, 2000.

Tierra, Lesley. *A Kid's Herb Book.* Brandon, OR: Robert D Reed Publishers, 2009.

Tierra, Lesley. *Healing with Chinese Herbs.* Freedom, CA: The Crossing Press, 1997.

Tierra, Lesley. *Healing with the Herbs of Life.* Berkeley, CA: The Crossing Press, 2003.

Tierra, Michael. *The Way of Chinese Herbs.* New York: Pocket Books, 1998.

Tierra, Michael. *The Way of Herbs.* New York: Pocket Books, 1998.

Tillotson, Alan Keith with Nai-shing Hu Tillotson and Robert Abel, Jr. *The One Earth Herbal Source Book: Everything You Need to Know about Chinese, Western, and Ayurvedic Herbal Treatments.* New York: Kensington Publishing, 2001.

Winston, David and Steven Maimes. *Adaptogens: Herbs for Strength, Stamina, and Stress Relief.* Rochester, VT: Healing Arts Press, 2007

Cookbooks

Bittman, Mark. *Leafy Greens.* Hoboken, NJ: Wiley Publishing, 2012.

Bittman, Mark. *How to Cook Everything Vegetarian.* Hoboken, NJ: Wiley Publishing, 2007.

Chuang, Lily. *Chinese Vegetarian Delights: Sugar and Dairy Free Cookbook.* Los Angeles: 7 Star Communications, 1987.

Chuang, Lily and Cathy McNease. *101 Vegetarian Delights.* Los Angeles: 7 Star Communications, 1992.

Colbin, Annemarie. *The Book of Whole Meals.* New York: Ballantine Books, 1985.

Credicott, Tammy. *Paleo Indulgences.* Las Vegas: Victory Belt Publishing, 2012.

Davis, William. *Wheat Belly Cookbook.* New York: Rodale, 2013.

Erhart, Shep and Leslie Cerier. *Sea Vegetable Celebration*. Summertown, TN: Book Publishing Co, 2001.

Gusman, Jill. *Vegetables from the Sea*. New York: Harper Collins Publishing, 2003.

Gyngell, Skye. *A Year in My Kitchen*. Berkeley, CA: 10 Speed Press, 2006.

Haas, Elson M. *The New Detox Diet: The Complete Guide for Lifelong Vitality with Receipes, Menus, & Detox Plans*. Berkeley, CA: Celestial Arts, 2004.

Kafka, Barbara with Christopher Styler. *Vegetable Love*. New York: Workman Publishing, 2005.

Katzen, Mollie. *The Heart of the Plate*. New York: Houghton, Mifflin, Harcourt, 2013.

Kaufmann, Doug and Denni Dunham. *Cooking Your Way to Good Health*. Rockwall, TX: Media Trition, 2011.

Lappe, Frances Moore. *Diet for a Small Planet*. New York: Ballantine Books, 1991.

Leggett, Daverick. *Recipes for Self-Healing*. Totnes, England: Meridian Press, 1999.

Madison, Deborah. *Local Flavors: Cooking and Eating from America's Farmer's Markets*. New York: Broadway Books, 2002.

Madison, Deborah. *Vegetable Soups from Deborah Madison's Kitchen*. New York: Broadway Books, 2006.

Natali, Nadia. *The Blue Heron Ranch Cookbook*. Berkeley, CA: North Atlantic Books, 2008.

Ody, Penelopy. *The Chinese Herbal Cookbook: Healing Foods for Inner Balance*. Trumbull, CT: Weatherhill, 2001.

Oliver, Jamie. *Jamie's 15 Minute Meals*. New York: Penguin Group, 2012.

Pickarski, Brother Ron. *Friendly Foods*. Berkeley, CA: Ten Speed Press, 1991.

Robertson, Laurel, Carol Flinders, and Brian Ruppenthal. *The New Laurel's Kitchen*. Berkeley, California: Ten Speed Press, 1986.

Simonds, Nina. *A Spoonful of Ginger*. New York: Alfred A Knopf, 1999.

Turner, Lisa. *Meals That Heal*. Rochester, VT: Healing Arts Press, 1996.

Watson, Ric and Trudy Thelander. *The Mediterrasian Way*. Hoboken, NJ: Wiley Publications, 2007.

Weil, Andrew, Sam Fox and Michael Stebner. *True Food*. New York: Little, Brown, and Co, 2012.

For Head and Heart

Brown, Brene. *Daring Greatly*. New York: Gotham Books, 2012.

Brown, Brene. *The Gifts of Imperfection*. Center City, MN: Hazelden, 2010.

Chodron, Pema. *Taking the Leap: Freeing Ourselves from Old Habits and Fears*. Boston: Shambhala, 2009.

Chodron, Pema. *The Pema Chodron Collection*. New York: One Spirit, 1991.

Crow, David. *In Search of the Medicine Buddha*. New York: Penguin Putnam, 2000.

Dalai Lama and Victor Chan. *The Wisdom of Forgiveness*. New York: Riverhead Books, 2004.

Grandin, Temple and Catherine Johnson. *Animals Make Us Human*. New York: Houghton Mifflin Harcourt, 2009.

Horowitz, Alexandra. *On Looking*. New York: Scribner, 2013.

Keville, Kathy and Mindy Green. *Aromatherapy: A Complete Guide to the Healing Art*. Freedom, CA: The Crossing Press, 1995.

Ni, Hua-Ching. *The Complete Works of Lao Tzu*. Los Angeles: 7 Star Communications, 1998.

Northrup, Christiane. *The Wisdom of Menopause*. New York: Bantam Books, 2006.

Ross, Julia. *The Mood Cure*. New York: Penguin Books, 2002.

Tzu, Lao. *The Tao Te Ching*. New translation by Ralph Alan Dale. London: Watkins Publishing, 2006.

Tolle, Eckhart. *A New Earth: Awakening to Your Life's Purpose*. New York: Penguin Group, 2006.

Tolle, Eckhart. *The Power of Now*. Novato, CA: Nameste Publishing, 1999.

Weil, Andrew. *Healthy Aging*. New York: Alfred A Knopf, 2005.

SOURCES FOR PURE ESSENTIAL OILS
1) *Floracopeia* Aromatic Treasures can be purchased at floracopeia.com.

2) *Snow Lotus* Artisan Essential Oils can be purchased at snowlotus.org.

3) *Simplers Botanicals* sells essential oils and herbs at simplers.com

SOURCES FOR HERBAL PRODUCTS

4) *Mayway* sells a variety of Chinese herbal products at mayway.com.

2) *Starwest Botanicals* sells mostly Western herbs, with some Chinese herbs at starwest-botanicals.com.

3) *Wild Rose Herbs* sells Western, Chinese and Ayurvedic herbs at wildro-seherbs.com.

About the Author

Cathy McNease holds a Diplomate in Chinese Herbology from the NCCAOM, a B.S. in Biology and Psychology from Western Michigan University and two Master Herbalist certificates from Emerson College of Herbology in Canada and East-West Course of Herbology in Santa Cruz. She has co-authored two books, *The Tao of Nutrition* and *101 Vegetarian Delights* and a distance learning course, *TCM Nutrition*. In addition to her teaching profession she maintains a Chinese herbal pharmacy business, Best Blends Herbs, and is in private practice in Santa Barbara and Ojai. She is a Professional Member of the American Herbalist Guild. Cathy has been an avid gardener for several decades with particular interest in growing medicinal and fragrant plants, as well as beautiful flowers.